Ask the Doctor
Breast Cancer

W9-BNK-851

by
Vincent Friedewald, M.D.
Coauthored by
Aman U. Buzdar, M.D.

Professor of Medicine and Deputy Chairman,
Breast Cancer Oncology Department
The University of Texas M. D. Anderson Cancer Center
Houston, Texas

with Michael Bokulich

Andrews and McMeel

A Universal Press Syndicate Company

Kansas City

Library of Congress Cataloging-in-Publication Data

Friedewald, Vincent E., 1941–
    Ask the doctor : Breast cancer / Vince
Friedewald and Aman U. Buzdar.
        p.   cm.
    ISBN 0–8362–2710–7 (pbk.)
    1. Breast—Cancer—Popular works.   I. Buzdar,
Aman U.   II. Title.
RC280.B8F738   1997
616.99´449—dc21   96–51957
                                                      CIP

Contents

Provided through an unrestricted
educational grant from
Zeneca Pharmaceuticals.

Foreword

You have been told that you have breast cancer.

You—not your neighbor, or the woman at work, or someone you went to school with.

Yes, it's you.

The word *cancer* carries with it a variety of emotions: fear, anger, bewilderment, feeling out of control. It seemed the world stopped when you first heard your diagnosis. And when the world started spinning again, you realized that your world would be different—at least for a while.

Your days would be filled with physician appointments, surgery, recovery, further treatment, radiation therapy, maybe chemotherapy. And there would be strange sensations in your breast, fatigue—sheer, deep, overwhelming fatigue—many questions, some answers, and more questions.

Getting answers to your questions and being completely informed about your breast cancer and your treatment plan allow you to feel in control again. Information is a powerful tool, as it helps explain the many things that are happening to you. It removes some of the fear and bewilderment.

And it provides you with information to tell others who are important to you—your spouse, friends, children, parents, sisters, or brothers. Information you provide can set them at ease and help restore the "usual" in all of your lives again.

Ask the Doctor: Breast Cancer is a comprehensive guide to breast cancer and its treatment. It is written for you, based on the experience of hundreds of women who are living "well" with breast cancer. You can use the book any way you like. Read it in order from beginning to end, or read only the chapters that meet your immediate needs.

The book's opening chapter addresses the question, "What Is Breast Cancer?" This chapter describes the changes that occur in the breast cell that allow it to become a cancer cell. It tells about the different types of breast cancer and emphasizes that body cells and breast cells are unique to each individual, and that *breast cancer differs from woman to woman*. Chapter 2 tells how breast cancer is diagnosed and explains the process, from mammography to ultrasound to biopsy.

Chapter 3 describes the importance of the treatment plan and stresses that the plan for each woman is specific. In other words, each treatment plan is different and based on such things as the type of cancer, the cancer stage, and the woman herself. It is important to understand your treatment plan and not to compare it with the treatment plan of others. Other women who have experienced breast cancer can provide great support, but please, *remember to use your doctor and nurse as the primary sources of information about your breast cancer.*

Chapters 4 through 7 walk you through the components of therapy: surgery, radiation, chemotherapy, and hormonal therapy. It is important to understand each of the components. These chapters should be read prior to starting each component of the treatment plan and as many times as needed while experiencing that component of the plan. Remember, each woman's treatment plan is "her" plan and may contain all or just some of the components described in the book. Be sure to ask your doctor or nurse if you have questions about "your" treatment plan.

Chapter 8 asks "How Are You Doing?" Just as each treatment plan is different, so is the reaction of each woman to her particular plan. Breast cancer and its treatment bring many emotional as well as physical issues and concerns. This is a time when you *need* support from others—your family, your physician and nurse, friends, other women who have had breast cancer. Accept the help and support others want to give, and read and learn all that you can. Use the information in this chapter to help cope with the ups and downs of breast cancer treatment and to help your family and friends with questions they may have. Try some of the helpful hints described in Chapter 8, but just as before, ask your doctor or nurse if you have questions.

Live each day to its fullest—rest and recover—accept the help of others—learn all that you can. Put one foot in front of the other, and walk through your treatment until you hear the magic words: "This is your last treatment." Even those long-anticipated words, though music to your ears, also bring new questions and fears: Will the treatment work? Will you become cancer-free? As Chapter 9 explains, some women require only the completion of one course of treatment, but others need retreatment once or several times. Again, each woman is different.

After the treatment is complete, the most important thing is to continue follow-up care with your doctor, and to follow the guidelines he or she gives you. You may continue to have questions and concerns, but as always, call your doctor or nurse for the answers.

I have been privileged to know many hundreds of women living with breast cancer. The road you are now traveling is often difficult. You are learning many new things about yourself and others that will become an enduring source of strength and knowledge. Most important, you will learn to live each day to its fullest, discovering a life of happiness and depth that others can never know.

Joyce M. Yasko, R.N., Ph.D., F.A.A.N.
Associate Director
Clinical and Network Administration
University of Pittsburgh Cancer Institute

Icons

Throughout *Ask the Doctor*, you will see a number of icons, symbols in the margins of each page. The icons are a very quick reference guide to help you look up information you may want to get to quickly. For example, if you want to read only about lymph nodes in relation to breast cancer, you could page through *Ask the Doctor* and look for all the paragraphs with the icon. The same goes for all the topics listed below:

 Very important information, talk to your doctor

 Age-related topics, both elderly and young

 Breast exam, by yourself or a physician

 Biopsy

 Coping and support

 Cosmetic issues, appearance

 Chemotherapy

 Diet

 "Doctorspeak," medical terminology

 Estrogen, progesterone

 Exercise

 Family history, heredity

 Hormonal therapy

 Medical history, prior conditions

 It's your turn

 Job, housework

 Lymph nodes, including lymphedema

 Metastasis

 Pregnancy, fertility

 Recurrent cancer

 Radiation therapy

 Side effects related to therapy

 Sexuality

 Surgery

1

What Is Breast Cancer?

CANCER IS A disease in which abnormal cells multiply beyond the body's control. When enough of these cells—in the millions—have grown in one place, they form a tumor.

The tumor is the lump under the breast, the spot on the mammogram, that mysterious, hidden collection of cells gone awry.

Let's start by getting rid of some of the mysteries—first, surrounding cancer in general. Then, we'll turn our attention to breast cancer.

It Begins with a Cell

Cells are the smallest parts of our body that are complete, living units. One of the things that cells *normally* do is divide to form more cells exactly like themselves. They do it predictably—to repair damaged cells, to replace old ones, and to grow. Some cells, like blood cells, divide at a very rapid rate, *according to what the body needs.*

Cancer, a Latin word, from the Greek *karkinos*, meaning "crab." According to the ancient Greek physician Galen, cancer was so named because the swollen veins around the tumor looked like a crab's limbs. These were seen while examining tumors from women with breast cancer.

So how is this different from cancer? The difference is that cancer cells don't care what the body needs. And they won't stop when the body tells them to. They take on a life of their own, independent of the host they live in, to the point of destroying normal cells and even themselves.

But why?

We don't know all the answers, but lots of the pieces of the puzzle have been put in place. Let's look at what we know.

A Cell with Damaged DNA

When a cell becomes cancerous, several events take place, all involving its DNA.

DNA is the blueprint inside every cell in every plant and animal on earth that governs all things about the cell. It carries the code that determines every feature of our bodies, from the color of our eyes to the length of our toes. DNA is also the link with our family, the thing that makes us, for better or worse, like our parents, brothers and sisters, and every other human being.

But, as terrific as DNA is, it isn't perfect. It can be damaged, and sometimes that damage results in cancer.

How does DNA become damaged? Again, the complete answer isn't known—that's a key to erasing cancer from the planet. But we know of at least three ways that DNA can become abnormal:

1. In the process of normal cell division, something goes wrong—a mistake, like a piece of the DNA falls off. This sort of mistake is called a *mutation.* The result is a newly formed cell containing damaged DNA.

2. Something outside the cell, even outside the body itself, harms the DNA. Such an external factor is called a *carcinogen* (something that causes cancer). For example, you already know that cigarette smoke is a carcinogen. Other things known to harm DNA are radiation and sunlight.

3. Abnormal DNA can be inherited (passed on by Mom or Pop). That's why many cancers run in families.

But that's not the end of the DNA story. Just having damaged DNA alone in one cell isn't enough to cause cancer, because the body has developed ways to cope with abnormal DNA. The body runs a quality-control check on DNA via other genes, called *tumor-*

Cancer is defined by four conditions:

- Cancer originates from genetic changes to a single cell, which multiplies to form a line, or clone, of similar malignant cells *(clonality).*

- Growth of the malignant cells is not properly regulated by the normal biologic and physical influences in the cell or body *(autonomy).*

- There is a lack of normal, coordinated cell differentiation *(anaplasia).*

- Cancer cells, unlike normal cells, develop the ability to spread to and grow in other distant parts of the body *(metastasis).*

suppressor genes, like the *p53 gene.* DNA production is closely watched by p53, and when p53 is doing its job correctly, it steps in and halts the process if it senses abnormal DNA.

When cancer occurs, something has gone wrong with the p53 guardians, and the cancer cell, with its abnormal DNA, multiplies free of the body's control.

So how does breast cancer fit into this picture? Let's take a short anatomy lesson first, then we'll see.

Your Breasts—a Different View

> The breast is actually a modified sweat gland, one modified to produce milk.

The breast is a collection of glands and fatty tissue actually extending far beyond what you can see. Breast tissue runs from about the collarbone down to the lowest rib, and from the breastbone to the area under the arm. Although the size and shape of breasts vary widely from person to person, such physical differences have absolutely nothing to do with cancer.

In the center (more or less) of each breast is the *nipple,* and the darker-colored ring surrounding the nipple is the *areola.*

Beneath the skin, the breast is made up of several types of tissue. Mostly, it is fat, which gives size and shape to the breasts. Within this fatty tissue, the milk glands spread out in a wagon-wheel pattern. The *lobules* are groups of individual milk-forming glands, called bulbs or acini, and are like very small bunches of grapes. These lobules empty into the *ducts,* which are thin tubes that carry milk to the nipple.

Inside these lobules and ducts is where most breast cancers begin.

The breast also contains connective tissue called *fascia,* which covers the milk glands and supports them. There are *blood vessels,* which supply the breast with nutrients and oxygen, and *nerves,* which give it sensation.

Underneath each breast are two large, flat muscles, the *pectoralis* muscles, which help to move the arms, and under these muscles are the ribs.

Finally, running throughout the breast is a vast network of *lymphatic vessels,* which connect to three strings of lymph nodes: the axillary lymph nodes under the arm; the supraclavicular lymph nodes under the collarbone; and the parasternal lymph nodes (or internal mammary nodes) alongside the breastbone.

The purpose of the lymphatics is to drain fluid and debris from the breast tissue to the lymph nodes, sort of like the local housekeeper. From the lymph nodes, the bloodstream carries the lymph away to be broken down and removed from the body.

Now let's look at breast cancer.

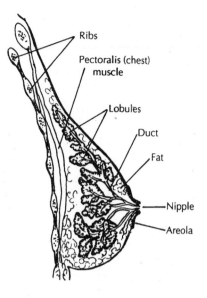

Ribs

Pectoralis (chest) muscle

Lobules

Duct

Fat

Nipple

Areola

When Does Breast Cancer Start?

Like other cancers, breast cancer starts with a single cell.

In the breast, that single cell is usually inside the lobules and ducts. Why there? Because that is where lots of cells normally divide during part of the menstrual cycle.

Each month, breast cells are signaled, by way of the hormones *estrogen* and *progesterone*, to begin dividing rapidly. This prepares the breasts for pregnancy and ultimately for breast-feeding. So the breasts swell. If pregnancy doesn't occur, a second signal is sent for the breast cells to stop multiplying, and the breasts shrink.

So every month, year after year, from the first onset of menses— called the *menarche*—to the end of menses—the *menopause*—this cycle of rapid cell growth inside the breasts repeats itself. And that raises the odds that a DNA mistake, a mutation, will occur sometime during those years.

That's when we believe that many breast cancers really begin, in the premenopausal years, even though most cancers usually aren't recognized until later in life.

And the estrogen and progesterone that stimulate the breast cells to grow during the monthly menstrual cycle also stimulate breast cancer cells, causing them to grow and divide more rapidly.

One more thing about these breast cancer cells: They tend to have "a mind of their own" and don't listen to the hormonal messages to stop dividing. They keep growing and multiplying, feasting on the estrogen. This will be important to remember later, when we discuss treatment.

> Cancers generally aren't noticed until the tumors are at least one half to one inch in size, which is about the size of a grape. Mammography can detect cancers about two years before they can be felt.

So a cancer may lie dormant or remain so small that it can't be felt or seen, even with the most sensitive tests, for many years. The cancer cells finally form a lump or mass, the *tumor*.

Genes and Breast Cancer

What role do genes play in breast cancer? Although the gene named *BRCA1* has received a lot of publicity, no single gene has been identified to be the sole culprit.

When *BRCA1* was isolated in late 1994, it was reported widely in the news as *the* cause of breast cancer. But then experts backed off, claiming that the gene was involved in only 5 percent of breast cancers—specifically a rarer form of inherited early-onset breast cancer. This type of breast cancer occurs in families, often striking women in their early thirties.

But most breast cancers (80 percent) occur in women over age fifty who do not have the defective *BRCA1* gene. Recently, experts have theorized that another, separate defect in *BRCA1* may be involved in these other cancers. A related gene, *BRCA2*, also has been associated with some breast cancers. And a third, *BRCA3*, is under study.

And what about the p53 gene that monitors for abnormal DNA? It's abnormal in 30 to 35 percent of breast cancer patients.

Many other genes have been found to be abnormal in women with breast cancer, but the same defects are not found in all. This is probably because cell growth is driven and controlled by many different genes and other factors. In fact, many different gene defects, working in different combinations, probably can cause cells to become cancerous.

Who Gets Breast Cancer?

In the same way that no one gene can account for all (or even most) breast cancers, likewise no single characteristic, or *risk factor*, can predict who will get breast cancer.

But we know that women who get breast cancer often have several things in common. Here are the ones best identified:

Well-established Risk Factors

Aging: The risk of developing breast cancer increases considerably with age. More than three-fourths of breast cancers develop in women who are over age fifty, and more than half occur in women age sixty-five and over. Yet, young women do get breast cancer, but less commonly. It is rare under age thirty.

No Prior Pregnancy: Being childless increases the risk for breast cancer by almost twice that of women who have had one or more babies. Abortion does not increase cancer risk, period.

Late Age of First Pregnancy: The later in life the first baby comes along, the higher the risk. And especially if it is delayed until after age thirty. The lowest risk is among women having their first child before age eighteen. Breast-feeding seems to have no effect.

Why is Early Birth Protective?
It is believed that the hormonal changes of pregnancy may cause breast tissue to "mature" and become resistant to cancerous transformation.

Family History: Breast cancer sometimes runs in families. If a mother, sister, or daughter—a "first-degree" relative—had breast cancer, then the risk is increased by one and a half to three times. That risk increases more if the relative's cancer developed before menopause or if it affected both breasts. But

What about *BRCA1*?
A defect in this gene is identified as causing hereditary, early-onset breast cancer. Among families carrying this gene, 85 percent of women might develop breast cancer in their lifetime, with 50 percent by age fifty. But this accounts for only a small number of women who get breast cancer, about 5 percent of the total. And not all breast cancers running in families are due to *BRCA1*. More research is needed before the true role of this gene is understood.

more than 70 percent of the women in these families will *not* develop breast cancer. And having aunts, cousins, and grandmothers with the disease increases the risk only slightly.

Higher Socioeconomic Status: Women with incomes in the upper two-thirds of the U.S. population get breast cancer more often than "poor" women. This may result from the tendency of women in higher-income groups to have children at a later age.

Early Menarche/Late Menopause: Earlier age at first menstruation (menarche before age twelve) and later cessation of menses (menopause after age fifty-five) increase the breast cancer risk. Why? Because more menstrual cycles take place, meaning more estrogen exposure and more opportunities for cells to become malignant.

Previous Cancer: Women who have had breast cancer before are at risk for a recurrence, both in the same and the opposite breast. Women who have had other cancers, including colon, uterine, or major salivary gland cancer and Hodgkin's disease, likewise face a higher risk of breast cancer.

Does Anything Reduce the Risk?

Many of the risk factors for breast cancer are items a woman can't do much about, like age of menarche, her genes, and, yes—even though men do occasionally get breast cancer— the female gender. A few actions are associated with a decreased risk:

- having a baby before age eighteen
- having the ovaries removed (oophorectomy) before age thirty-five
- having the breasts removed (prophylactic mastectomy)
- physical exercise

None of these eliminates the risk entirely, however.

"Premalignant" Diseases: Some types of breast disease, though not cancer, carry a slight risk for cancer to develop later. These conditions are detected by biopsy and include *atypical hyperplasia*, multiple *papillomatosis*, and certain forms of *large cystic disease*. However, fibrocystic disease of the breast does *not* carry increased risk.

More Risk Factors

Several more factors appear to *slightly* increase the risk for breast cancer, but their role is either unclear or very small—too small to worry about.

Alcohol: Alcohol consumption increases estrogen levels, so two or more drinks a day might increase the risk, especially in younger women.

Radiation Exposure: Exposure to ionizing radiation, especially for women under age thirty, can raise the risk for the later development of breast cancer. But radiation exposure doesn't happen often. And the doses used to detect breast cancer via mammography are safe.

Adult Weight Gain: Body fat produces estrogen, and that increase in circulating estrogen is an added risk in the post-menopausal woman.

DES: Women who took diethylstilbestrol (DES), an estrogenlike agent, while pregnant have a slightly increased chance of breast cancer in later years.

Oral Contraceptives: This risk is debatable. Most studies show no risk, but long-term use (more than ten years) or use at a very young age might increase the risk.

Lack of Physical Exercise: One study has shown that women under age forty who exercised at moderate amounts reduced their chances of breast cancer. This protective effect has not been proven for exercise at older ages.

Postmenopausal Estrogen Replacement

Short-term hormone replacement therapy (HRT) is safe, but because it puts estrogen back into the system, there is concern that the risk of breast cancer (as well as cancer of the uterus) may increase, especially if it is continued over ten to twenty years or if there is a strong history of breast (or uterine) cancer in the family. However, newer studies show no higher risk of breast cancer in postmenopausal women with no previous history of breast cancer who receive HRT. Furthermore, HRT has proven benefits in reducing cardiovascular disease, which is the leading cause of death in women, and osteoporosis (bone loss), which is the cause of thousands of bone fractures in older women every year.

Bottom line: The pluses and minuses of HRT should be discussed with a doctor—not friends and neighbors and daytime talk-show gurus—before making a decision about HRT.

Things That Don't Affect Risk

Diet: The high-fat Western diet has been blamed for increases in breast cancer, due mostly to the large difference seen in breast cancer rates between developed countries, with their rich, high-fat diets, and less-developed countries. But diet may not be the culprit here. Vegetarians and others in Western countries who eat a low-fat diet show similar rates as everyone else. And no specific diet or vitamin has been proven to *decrease* breast cancer risk either.

Fibrocystic Breasts: Fibrocystic breasts do not place a woman at higher risk for breast cancer. Likewise, other benign breast diseases—including cysts and infections—do not increase the risk.

Smoking: Smoking does not increase breast cancer risk, although it may interfere with the response to breast cancer treatments. However, it is a major cause of lung cancer, heart disease, and many other serious illnesses, which lead to far more deaths than breast cancer.

Abortion: Despite claims to the contrary, abortion does *not* affect breast cancer risk. A recent study, looking at the health records of the entire female population of Denmark, showed no relationship between any aspect of abortion and the later development of breast cancer.

Other Factors: As for breast-feeding, large breasts (or small breasts), silicone breast implants, breast injury, infection, caffeine, chocolate, bras, engine exhaust, food and water contaminants—they have no effect on risk for breast cancer. Pesticides, PCBs, powerlines, and microwaves are under study, but there is not yet evidence for any effect from these, either.

So much for the causes and the risks. Now, let's take a look at breast cancer itself.

There's More Than One Type

The first cell in the breast that turns cancerous is usually—80 percent of the time—a cell that lines the milk ducts. This type is called a *ductal* tumor.

Less often—about 10 percent of the time—breast cancer starts in one of the cells lining the milk-forming lobules, and it is called a *lobular* tumor.

In both types, the cancer is termed an *adenocarcinoma*, so the most common forms of breast cancer are ductal adenocarcinomas and lobular adenocarcinomas.

Breast tumors are further classified by some other characteristics, which basically describe how and where the tumor is growing. These distinctions, which affect treatment decisions, are made by a pathologist when examining a sample of cells from a breast *biopsy*, or surgically removed piece of tumor tissue.

Here are some descriptions of abnormal biopsy findings related to breast cancer.

Adenocarcinoma
The word's roots are *adeno-*, meaning it is related to a gland—like the mammary glands in the breasts—and *carcinoma*, meaning it is derived from a certain cell type, called an epithelial cell.

Ductal Carcinoma in Situ (DCIS)

DCIS is breast cancer at its earliest stage. *In situ* is a Latin term meaning that the tumor is confined "in place." It is located entirely within the ducts and has not penetrated the duct walls to invade the surrounding breast tissue. But DCIS is cancerous. And it may spread widely through the ducts, affecting a large area of the breast.

These tumors, also known as intraductal or noninvasive ductal carcinomas, usually are first found on mammograms as *microcalcifications*, which are little specks or dots of calcium. They rarely form lumps and cannot easily be found on physical examination.

DCIS may be subdivided into *comedo* and *noncomedo* varieties, the former being the more serious. DCIS accounts for about 10 percent of breast cancers.

Infiltrating Ductal Carcinoma

Cancers that penetrate the duct wall and enter the surrounding breast tissue are termed *invasive* or *infiltrating*. This is the most common type of breast cancer, accounting for about 80 percent of cases.

When the cancer enters the surrounding breast, it usually becomes encased in a shell of tough, scarlike material, forming the lump noted in the breast or on the mammogram.

Various types of this form of breast cancer are sometimes noted and include terms such as *comedocarcinoma*, *medullary*, *tubular*, *mucinous*, and *NOS* (not otherwise specified).

Infiltrating Lobular Carcinoma

Invasive lobular tumors, like the ductal variety, penetrate the lobule walls to invade the surrounding fatty breast tissue. They also become surrounded by a tough, fibrous shell, but instead of forming a lump, they send out finger-like projections that are difficult to feel on a breast exam.

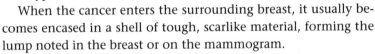

Male Breast Cancer

Men develop breast cancer too, though not very often. In the United States, about one thousand men per year develop it, which makes it less than 1 percent of all breast cancers. Like women, the men usually have invasive ductal carcinoma, and the treatment is basically the same.

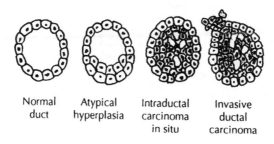

Normal duct   Atypical hyperplasia   Intraductal carcinoma in situ   Invasive ductal carcinoma

These tumors account for 5 to 10 percent of breast cancers and can cause simultaneous tumors in both breasts a bit more often than the ductal variety.

Other Types of Breast Cancer

Some rarer forms of breast cancer sometimes occur, including:

Inflammatory Breast Carcinoma: This form of breast cancer mimics an infection, appearing as an area of redness and warmth, like mastitis, but it does not clear up with antibiotics. *Peau d'orange* is a term sometimes used to describe the swollen appearance of the skin in this cancer.

Paget's Disease: Paget's disease of the nipple or breast starts with an itching, scaling rash on the nipple and areola *on only one breast*. There may be discharge or bleeding from the nipple.

Cystosarcoma Phyllodes: This unusual tumor is one of the least aggressive. It occurs in women who have fibroadenomas, which are large, recurrent, benign tumors. In rare cases, it can become malignant and behave like an aggressive cancer.

Other uncommon cancer types include *squamous cell carcinoma, angiosarcoma, lymphoma, carcinocarcinoma,* and *sweat gland carcinoma.*

Precancerous Conditions

Some breast changes, while not cancerous in themselves, are warning signs that cancer might develop at some point in the future:

Atypical Hyperplasia: This means that there is an over-growth of cells (hyperplasia) in the ducts or lobules, but it is not cancer. In a small percentage of women (10 to 20 percent), it may progress to cancer. Close follow-up for signs of developing cancer is advisable.

Lobular Carcinoma in Situ (LCIS): Whereas DCIS (ductal carcinoma in situ) affects the ducts, LCIS involves the milk-producing lobules. But unlike DCIS, LCIS isn't cancerous, though with time it may develop into cancer in about 25 percent of women. LCIS doesn't show up on mammograms. Its treatment is controversial.

Benign Breast Diseases

When the biopsy of a breast mass is "negative" (no cancer cells detected), one of several benign breast conditions might be reported as causing the mass:

- Breast cysts or cystic disease
- Fibrocystic disease
- Lipoma
- Fibroadenoma
- Infection
- Fat necrosis
- Intraductal papilloma
- Mammary duct ectasia
- Mondor's disease

Anyone having a breast biopsy should discuss it with the doctor and have a *clear understanding* of exactly what the results were, what they mean, and what follow-up is needed.

Obviously, a biopsy report that comes back negative does not mean the biopsy was unnecessary. Often, it is the only way to rule out the possibility of having breast cancer.

Tumor Spread

While the tumor is small and undetectable, it usually remains confined within one area of the breast. At that point, it is unlikely that the cancer has spread any farther.

When a tumor has grown to about half an inch in size and can be seen on a mammogram, local and distant spread is more likely. By the time a tumor is felt by self-examination, it measures one inch or more, and the chances of spread have increased even more.

Local or Regional Involvement

Local or *regional spread* refers to the spread of tumor directly into neighboring tissues. The tumor grows out in several directions in fingerlike projections and can involve multiple areas of the breast.

Tumors can also grow down to involve the chest muscles and ribs. Such tumors feel "fixed" to the underlying structures. Tumors may also grow outward to involve the skin.

And tumors can spread regionally via the lymphatic vessels. When this occurs, the lymph nodes under the arm (*axillary* nodes), alongside the breastbone (*internal mammary* nodes), or by the collarbone (*supraclavicular* nodes) may become enlarged.

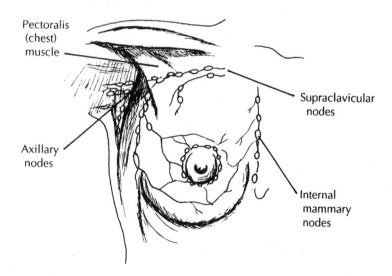

Pectoralis (chest) muscle

Supraclavicular nodes

Axillary nodes

Internal mammary nodes

Distant Metastasis

Metastasis refers to the distant spread of cancer to another site in the body. One way this happens is for the tumor cells in lymph glands to be picked up and spread by the bloodstream. New blood vessels (called *neovascularization*) typically form around a tumor, providing a new route for cancer cells to escape the tumor and enter the circulation.

The bone, liver, lung, and even the brain are typical sites for metastasis from breast cancer.

How Breast Cancer Destroys

But what is it about breast cancer that makes it so destructive? Several things:

- First is the various ways that it grows. One of these growth patterns is invasion. Breast cancer can grow into the chest wall and invade nearby organs, such as the liver or lung, interfering with their function.

  More commonly, breast cancer spreads by metastasis. Individual cells break off from the main tumor and travel to other parts of the body. Like seeds carried by the bloodstream or lymphatic fluid, the breast cancer cells take hold in distant sites and begin to grow, forming new tumors and causing loss of function in those distant organs as well.

- The second way that breast cancer harms the body is by competing with it for nutrients—sugar, proteins, minerals, even vitamins are needed to support the tumor's rapid growth.

- A third way is by putting the body's metabolism out of balance. For example, if breast cancer metastasizes to the bones, it can cause the release of calcium stored there. This raises the amount of calcium in the bloodstream, causing serious effects throughout the body.

- Finally, and often the most destructive effect of breast cancer, is what it does to the mind, even when not a single cancer cell has escaped a tiny area within the breast. Fear, depression, anxiety, and the resulting disruption it can have on the simplest tasks of daily life are, in many women, its most crippling effects.

Learning as much about breast cancer as you can and discussing each and every concern with your physician are important steps in helping you cope with this last effect.

Everyone's Different

You have heard of or seen women with breast cancer who have had remarkably easy recoveries. Others have had tragic experiences. Some get one form of treatment, others something completely different. And each person's response is so different.

That's because everyone's different!

And just as each person is unique, cancer tends to behave differently in each person too. There are many factors playing a role in the development and growth of a tumor, and an infinite number of variations are possible.

So what's the point? Just this: If you have breast cancer, it's easy to get confused by lots of advice from well-meaning friends and relatives who try to apply their "expertise" to you.

We designed this book to help you with answers to some of the many questions that will arise, based on the most recent expert opinion available.

But the fact is, the only person who can give you the best information is your doctor, because only your doctor knows you and your cancer. *That's the one person you should rely on for advice, for guidance, and for ultimate success.*

It's Your Turn

1. Has breast cancer occurred in any family members?
   ❏   Mother
   ❏   Sister
   ❏   Daughter
   ❏   Grandmother
   ❏   Aunt
   ❏   Other: _____

2. When did you first notice the lump or other suspicious finding?
   ❏   Found on mammography
   ❏   Within the last 2 weeks
   ❏   Within the last 2 months
   ❏   Longer? How long? _____

3. How large is the lump?
   ❏   1/2 inch (1 centimeter)
   ❏   1 inch (2–3 cm)
   ❏   2 inches (5 cm)

4. Are any lymph nodes swollen?
   ❏   Yes
   ❏   No
Where? _____

5. If you have had a biopsy and breast cancer was found, you should know the pathologist's description of the tumor. Write it here:

_____

2

Making the Diagnosis

IF YOU'VE FOUND a lump—or for any other reason you are concerned that you may have breast cancer—what should you do next?

First, if you haven't seen a doctor, make an appointment *now*. Most women start with their family physician or gynecologist. If you don't have a regular doctor, try the local women's health services or call a hospital referral service for a recommendation.

But first, exactly what sort of lump or other things about your breast should concern you?

Causes of Suspicion

There are several suspicious symptoms or findings that should be reported to a physician for evaluation:

- A lump or thickening in or near the breast or underarm area
- Unusual change in size or shape of the breast (swelling)
- Change in the color or feel of the skin on the breast (dimpled, puckered, thickened, scaly, or redness)
- Bloody discharge from the nipple, or scaly skin on the nipple or areola
- Inversion of the nipple

Let's take a closer look at these.

Lumps

The first sign of breast cancer is usually a lump. Most often, it is found by the woman herself. It also may be discovered by a physician in the course of a regular physical examination or on a mammogram.

With breast cancer, there is typically one lump in one breast. It is firm or hard and is seldom painful. Its size can range from tiny and barely detectable, even to an experienced examiner's hands, up to a visible bulge several inches across.

Now, almost every woman has found a lump in her breast at some time. And it can be difficult for you and your doctor to decide if it is an abnormal growth.

Not All Lumps Are Really Lumps
How can you tell if it really is a lump that you feel? Remember, many breast changes are normal. Breasts change with your menstrual cycle, and they change over your lifetime. The best solution is to practice regular breast self-examination so that you can come to know what your breasts feel like normally. Then, you'll know much better what changes should arouse concern.

Breasts are naturally "lumpy" in many women because of the many glands they contain. Doctors sometimes refer to these as *fibrocystic* breasts. Often, the lumpiness is more noticeable in the week before your period, but then subsides with your period.

In general, lumps are common in younger, premenopausal women. So, for younger women, the doctor may choose to reexamine you in several weeks, to see if the lump changes after your period. When a lump remains constant in size throughout the menstrual cycle or over a period of time, it becomes more suspect as a tumor.

After menopause, when the milk glands have shrunk, lumps due to normal cyclic changes in the breasts are much less common and should be checked more carefully.

In some women, though, breast cancer doesn't appear first as a lump. Instead, something else may arouse suspicion, including:

Bloody Discharge from the Nipple

Usually, bleeding from the nipple is caused by a noncancerous condition, such as an infection or even a small benign tumor in the duct. But it should always be checked by a doctor, because cancer can be the cause.

Skin or Nipple Changes

Breast cancer can sometimes cause an unusual skin thickening in one area of the breast, dimpling or puckering of the skin, or a scaly rash over part of one breast. A recent change in the size or shape of one breast or a nipple that suddenly becomes inverted (if it hasn't always been that way) is also suspicious.

These are uncommon signs of breast cancer. But if they occur, it is essential to have them checked by a doctor, just as a lump should be examined.

Seeing the Doctor

By now, you no doubt get the picture—see a doctor when there is any reason to suspect breast cancer. Waiting is a dangerous game, even when it turns out that cancer is not present.

Your History

During your visit, the doctor will ask a series of questions, but don't be embarrassed to admit if you don't know any or all the answers:

- How long has the lump been present?
- Has it changed over the course of the month (with your menstrual cycle)?

- Has breast cancer occurred in other family members, such as a mother or sister?

And, of course, you will be asked about your general medical and reproductive history.

The Physical Exam

The doctor will examine both of your breasts and the surrounding areas of your chest.

The breast exam has two parts, one in the sitting position, then lying down. First, the doctor looks at the skin and shape of each breast, checking for rashes, swellings, and lumps. Next, the doctor palpates your breasts to find the lump and, if there is one, to compare it with other areas of your breasts. Other areas, especially the underarm where key lymph nodes are grouped, will also be carefully examined.

The doctor's main purpose at this time is to check for what's called a "dominant" lump—a firm, single lump that feels unlike other breast tissue. The lump's size, texture, borders, and whether it is easily movable are all important. Swollen lymph nodes are another suspicious finding, especially if they are hard or "fixed."

Sometimes, a doctor can't be sure about a lump based on one examination, especially in younger women. He or she may decide to wait for a few weeks and then reexamine you, to see if the lump changes with your period. If you are older, especially if you are post-menopausal, when breast cancer is more common, the doctor may elect to order a mammogram or biopsy after just one exam.

Remember, even though lumps are usually benign, some prove to be cancer, and it's important to proceed with additional tests if that's what the doctor advises.

The Mammogram

A mammogram is a low-dose X ray of the breast. It shows the exact location of the lump, its shape, and certain features that point for or against cancer. It also detects any additional possible cancer sites in the breasts, even though they cannot be felt.

For this, you will be sent to a mammography center or other facility that specializes in radiology. (Radiology is the medical field that uses X rays to record images of your body's tissues and organs.)

The mammogram does not shrink or cure breast cancer. Nor does it cause tumors or make them worse. It is only a *very* important diagnostic aid.

How Should You Prepare?

There are no special precautions about eating or drinking before a mammogram. Dressing in a shirt that is easy to remove, rather than a dress or pullover, will be more convenient.

Avoid wearing jewelry, and avoid using deodorant or talcum powder because the dust may interfere with the X rays.

If you have copies of previous mammograms in your possession, take them with you to the radiologist for comparison.

Having a Mammogram

For the procedure, you will be asked to remove your shirt and bra and all jewelry. The technician places your bare breast on top of a plastic or metal plate that is attached to the mammography machine. She then lowers a top plate that presses against your breast, squeezing it. This pressure may be uncomfortable, but not painful. The pressure from the plate spreads out the breast so that masses are more easily visible and so that a lower dose of X rays can be used. This is repeated for the other breast.

The procedure itself is fairly simple and takes only a few minutes. For screening, two views are usually taken *in each breast*—a top view and a side view. More views may be taken when a lump has already been found or if there has been prior breast surgery, such as breast implants.

Before you leave, the radiologist will check the films quickly to make sure that they are satisfactory for all the questions the mammogram is designed to answer. Sometimes, additional X rays will need to be obtained before you leave.

The radiologist later studies the X rays more carefully and sends a report to your doctor, usually in a day or two. And remember, it is important that *you* be given a complete report, even if it is normal, for future reference.

Uncle Sam Cares

In 1992, Congress passed a law to license all facilities that perform mammography. Before this, mammograms sometimes were done by inexperienced operators or facilities with poor equipment. Since this law took effect in late 1994, these problems have been improved. To be licensed, every facility must meet standards for its equipment and show that its staff are properly trained.

What Exactly Does the Mammogram Show?

An X ray is like the negative of a photograph. The breast tissue and fat show up as pale gray. The ducts are fine white lines, like cotton candy. What about the questionable mass or lump? Here are some of the features the radiologist looks for:

- If a mass appears on the mammogram as smooth and round, it may be a simple cyst.

- *Microcalcifications*, which are little white specks of calcium, may be present. If these are spread out, they are probably normal, but if clustered in a small area or in a line, they add to the suspicion for cancer.

- If the outline of the breast is distorted, it could mean there is a tumor or growth pushing the normal tissue aside.

- An odd-shaped white spot or starburst-shaped spot is very suspicious for cancer.

As valuable as the mammogram is, it still doesn't give the final word on whether a lump is cancerous or not. So, if a lump looks suspicious on the mammogram, other tests are needed.

And not all lumps show up on the mammogram, either. Younger women tend to have denser breasts with more ducts and glands, sometimes making it harder to see a lump with this method. So, if a lump is felt but cannot be seen on the mammogram, other tests still may be necessary.

Finally, if you feel certain that you have a lump, and the mammogram doesn't show one, be sure to discuss it with your doctor—and thor- *oughly understand what should be done next.* Until all doubt has been removed, the matter should not be put off or dropped, regardless of whether additional tests are recommended.

Ultrasound and Other Imaging Tests

Another test that is sometimes performed is an *ultrasound* or *sonogram*. This test beams harmless and painless sound waves (which you cannot hear) into your breasts, where the waves are reflected back to form an image of the structures inside. Although ultrasound is not absolutely definitive about whether a mass is truly a cancer, it is very good in showing if a lump is a hollow, fluid-filled cyst (benign).

Two other "imaging" techniques also are occasionally done during diagnosis, primarily in research settings. *Magnetic resonance imaging* (MRI) and *positron emission tomography* (PET) both may provide useful information in younger patients, in whom the denser breast tissue can make mammograms unclear.

The Biopsy

When the mammogram (or ultrasound) fails to convince your doctor that a lump is not cancer, the next step is a biopsy.

This involves removing a sample of tissue or cells from the lump, either with a special needle or through a small surgical procedure. This sample is then given to a *pathologist*, who uses a microscope to study the cells for signs of cancer. Only a small piece of the breast is removed during biopsy, leaving only a small scar, if any.

Most Biopsies Rule Out Cancer

The huge majority of women who have biopsies turn out to have benign (noncancerous) results. For every five or ten women who are biopsied because of findings suspicious for breast cancer, only one is actually found to have cancer.

Let's look at the two types of biopsies, *needle* and *surgical*.

Needle Biopsy

Fine-needle aspiration biopsy uses a thin, hollow needle attached to a syringe. The procedure may be performed in the doctor's office. After a local anesthetic is applied to the breast, a needle is inserted into the lump and a sample of fluid or cells is withdrawn.

If the lump is a cyst, a clear or yellow fluid will be withdrawn, causing the cyst to collapse. This may be the only treatment needed for cysts, which are benign, although the doctor might want to follow up later to see if the cyst recurs.

If the fluid withdrawn is blood-tinged, if the lump turns out to be solid, or if the laboratory detects abnormal cells, then a surgical biopsy may be required for more testing.

Other needle biopsy techniques may be used on occasion. In a *core needle biopsy*, also called *core-cut biopsy*, a thicker needle is inserted into the lump, and a larger sample of tissue is removed for examination. If the lump is small or hard to reach, or if it is seen on X rays but cannot be felt, a technique called *stereotactic aspiration* may be used, in which mammograms are used to direct the needle into the tumor.

Many lumps are simply too deep or otherwise can't be reached with a needle, and a surgical biopsy is required in those instances.

Surgical Biopsy

Surgical biopsy removes a larger piece of the lump than needle biopsy, allowing for a better examination by the pathologist. *It is the only sure way to tell if a lump is really cancerous.* In a few instances, a surgical biopsy may be ordered even before a mammogram is done.

The biopsy is done by a surgeon, usually at a day surgery center or as an outpatient in the office. A local anesthetic is used, along with a calming sedative, so the patient remains awake during the procedure but doesn't feel pain.

The procedure lasts less than an hour, and you are sent home shortly after it is completed. The breast will be sore and a bit bruised, but only a small scar will result.

If the lump is small, a *lumpectomy* or *excisional biopsy* may be done. In this, the entire lump is removed in one procedure and is then sent to the pathologist. This approach combines both diagnosis (biopsy) and treatment in one operation, because if the lump is cancerous, no further surgery is required—although radiation, chemotherapy, and/or hormonal therapy will be. The doctor may also biopsy some of the lymph nodes under the arm to see if cancer has spread to these areas. (See Chapter 4 for more on breast-conserving surgery.)

For larger lumps, only a section of the tumor can be removed for testing. This is called an *incisional biopsy*. If cancer is found, more surgery will be planned later to remove the remaining tumor. Radiation and other treatment also will follow.

Sometimes, if the lump is too small to be felt, a special biopsy

A Better Way

In the past, biopsy was often part of a *one-step procedure*. In this, under general anesthesia, a biopsy was followed immediately by mastectomy in the same operation if cancer was found in the biopsy specimen. Since 1979, the National Cancer Institute has recommended a *two-step procedure* in which the biopsy is first performed, followed by surgery, if needed, at a later time. This approach gives the patient an opportunity to discuss treatment options as well as time to begin the emotional adjustment to the consequences of cancer and surgery.

technique called a *wire-localization biopsy* may be carried out. In this procedure, mammograms are used to direct a small wire into the tumor. The wire guides the surgeon to the tumor, who then performs a regular surgical biopsy.

The Pathology Report

After the biopsy, the pathologist sends a report describing the findings to the doctor. This includes the results of special tests performed on the tumor tissue that are important in determining which treatment will be best for the specific tumor.

The most important aspects of the report are the tumor size, extent of lymph node involvement (more on this in Chapter 4), tumor grade, and whether the tumor is positive for hormone receptors.

- *Size*—Tumor size is noted in centimeters (cm).

- *Tumor type*—Whether the cancer is intraductal or intralobular, in situ or invasive, and any subtype (these types are discussed in Chapter 1).

- *Margins*—These refer to the edges of a tumor. If the margins are "clean," the tumor was well-contained and probably removed in full. Otherwise, tumor cells might have spread outside the portion of breast tissue that was removed. Therefore, additional surgery, radiotherapy, or chemotherapy will be needed to kill the remaining cancer.

- *Vascular or lymphatic involvement*—Tumors that grow into blood vessels or lymphatics are considered more likely to have spread.

- *Hormone receptor assays*—Tumors are called *estrogen receptor (ER)–positive* or *progesterone receptor (PR)–positive* if they carry extra receptors for these hormones, which may stimulate cancer cell growth. Tumors that are ER-positive tend to respond better to hormonal treatment (see Chapter 7) and are more common in postmenopausal women.

- *Grade*—A score according to the appearance of the tumor cells. More normal-appearing cells, Grade I, tend to be less aggressive. Grade III is more severe and is the most common grade.

- *Ploidy and S-phase*—A technique called flow cytometry is used to tell whether extra chromosomes are present in the cells (aneuploidy) and how many cells are in a rapid growth phase (S-phase). When present, either of these phases indicates a more aggressive tumor.

Tumor Markers

Tumor cells sometimes produce "markers" as evidence of rapid cell division or growth, implying a need for more aggressive treatment. These markers are largely research tools and the list is much longer than the few noted here:

    p53

    nm23

    HER2/neu/c-erbB-2

    epidermal growth factor (EGF)

    angiogenesis factor (new blood vessel growth)

More Tests

If cancer is found, treatment usually begins within a few weeks after the biopsy has been obtained. Before treatment starts, some studies are performed to assess the woman's general health and condition and to search for distant spread (metastasis) of the cancer. If not already performed, these studies may include:

- *A complete history*
- *Physical examination*—to check for swollen lymph nodes, skin changes suggesting possible spread, and liver involvement
- *Pelvic examination*—to check for uterine cancer
- *Blood tests*—including a complete blood count, liver and kidney function tests, and calcium and phosphorus levels

CEA, or *carcinoembryonic antigen*, is a tumor marker that appears in blood when people have cancer. Levels of this marker can change, so measuring it may be useful in judging a response after therapy. Another tumor marker found in blood is CA 15-3, and it also may be measured to follow the progress of treatment.

And More X Rays

Depending on the size of the tumor and some other signs, more radiologic tests may be needed before treatment starts. These "imaging" studies check for the spread of cancer to bones and other organs, such as the liver and brain.

- *Chest X ray*—to check for spread to the lungs and to the ribs and spine.

- *Liver scan*—a CAT scan, or computed tomography, to evaluate the liver, especially if the liver tests suggest metastasis to that organ. CAT scans of the brain and lungs are also sometimes performed, depending on other findings in the evaluation.

- *Bone scan*—to rule out spread of cancer to the bone. Often, this test isn't necessary with small cancers.

It's Your Turn

1. Does the lump change with your period?
   - ❏   Yes
   - ❏   No

2. How long has the lump been there?
   - ❏   1 month
   - ❏   2–3 months
   - ❏   Longer? How long? _____

3. If you had a mammogram, what did it show?
   - ❏   Nothing unusual; All clear*
   - ❏   Unclear; the doctor can't tell*
   - ❏   Microcalcifications
   - ❏   A large cluster or multiple areas of abnormal findings

*If you can feel a lump but it doesn't show on the mammogram, more tests are needed.

4. Which kind of biopsy did you have?
   - ❑ Needle aspiration
   - ❑ Excisional or lumpectomy
   - ❑ Incisional
   - ❑ Special technique: _____

5. What type of tumor is it?
   Ductal _____ *or* lobular _____
   In situ _____ *or* invasive _____
   What subtype? _____

6. How large is the tumor?
   - ❑ 1 cm or less (less than $1/2$ inch, pea-sized)
   - ❑ 2 cm ($3/4$ inch, a grape)
   - ❑ 3 cm ($1 1/4$ inches, a Ping-Pong ball)
   - ❑ 4 cm ($1 1/2$ inches, a golf ball)
   - ❑ 5 cm (2 inches, a tennis ball)

7. Is the tumor positive or negative for hormone receptors?
   - ❑ ER-positive *or* ❑ ER-negative
   - ❑ PR-positive *or* ❑ PR-negative

8. If you have had any of these tests, what did they show?
   - ❑ Complete physical and history
   - ❑ Blood tests
   - ❑ Pelvic (gynecologic) exam
   - ❑ Chest X ray
   - ❑ Liver scans*
   - ❑ Bone scans*

*Not always necessary, especially with smaller tumors.

3

What Course of Treatment?

Aᴦᴛᴇʀ ᴛʜᴇ ʙɪᴏᴘsʏ, surgical removal of the tumor is usually the first step in treatment, followed by other forms of therapy over a period of several weeks to months. Your first reaction might be to have the surgery right away. But there is no reason to rush if you need time to consider your options. You can take a few weeks to gather information to better understand your particular situation and the treatment alternatives.

During this time you may encounter friends or other women who have had breast cancer, and you may discover a variety of ways others have been treated. That's because breast cancer truly differs from woman to woman. Furthermore, treatment today is very different from the approach someone else may have experienced only a few years ago.

For example, in the not so distant past, women were usually given one option for treating breast cancer: a *radical mastectomy*, which is total removal of the breast and surrounding tissues. This, of course, wasn't really an option at all; this drastic surgery was *just done,* because that's what doctors used to believe was needed to bring about a cure. Since then, we have learned that most forms of breast cancer do not require such extensive surgery. In most cases, more limited, breast-conserving surgery has equally effective results.

So what are the different treatments, and how are they selected?

Assessing the Tumor

The best course of treatment is based on a number of factors that we've outlined below. But remember, *your views and desires are very important in this planning.* So ask plenty of questions and understand exactly what's being recommended and why. And make sure your doctor understands your views and concerns before proceeding.

Staging

Staging is one of the methods doctors use to decide the right treatment plan.

The stage of breast cancer is determined by two things: the size of the tumor and whether it has spread outside the breast. The stage is one measure of how severe the cancer is.

There are five stages:

- *Stage 0:* This is the earliest type of breast cancer. The cancer is said to be "in situ," or confined to the ducts or lobules. It has not invaded the surrounding breast tissue. There are two varieties, lobular carcinoma in situ (LCIS) and ductal carcinoma in situ (DCIS). LCIS is not really cancer yet and instead is considered a marker that cancer might develop someday in the future (which it will in 25 percent of women having LCIS). DCIS, however, is definitely cancer.

- *Stage I:* There is a tumor, but it is less than one inch in diameter and has not spread outside the breast.

- *Stage II:* The tumor is about one to two inches in diameter and may have spread to the lymph nodes under the arm (the axillary lymph nodes). It is further divided into two subtypes, *A* and *B,* depending mostly on whether the lymph nodes are involved.

- *Stage III:* This cancer is called *locally advanced.* The tumor is large, about two inches or more in diameter, and has spread to the surrounding lymph nodes or other tissues near the breast. There are two subtypes. In *Stage IIIA,* the tumor has spread to the axillary lymph nodes under the arm. In *Stage IIIB,* it involves the nearby tissues, such as the skin, chest muscles, ribs, or the lymph nodes along the breastbone.

- *Stage IV:* This is metastatic cancer. The cancer has spread beyond the breast and local lymph nodes and into other organs of the body. The lung, liver, and bone are the most common sites of metastases.

Inflammatory breast carcinoma, which is a relatively rare type of breast cancer, is considered as a separate class, but it is treated as Stage IIIB.

TNM System Made Simple

The system doctors use to assign a stage is called the TNM system, and it is a little complicated. *T* stands for tumor and describes the tumor's size and local invasion. *N* stands for nodes, which indicates if the tumor has spread to the lymph nodes around the breast. *M* is metastasis, or spread to other organs. Each of these letters also has a number with it, referring to if and how much these are involved—for instance, 0 means none, 1 means some, and 2 means more, and so on. So, T1N1M0 means a small tumor less than one inch in size, with evidence of cancer in the underarm lymph nodes, and no spread to other organs—Stage IIA, highly treatable.

Menopausal Status

The choice of treatment also depends on whether a woman has passed the menopause. Women who are postmenopausal tend to have breast tumors that contain estrogen hormone receptors, making them likely to respond to hormonal therapy. Women who are premenopausal often do not have these hormone receptors in their tumors and may require chemotherapy.

Hormone Receptors

Breast cancer cells often contain a huge number of chemical "receptors," or sites that attract the body hormones estrogen and progesterone. These hormones stimulate the cancer cells to grow faster. Tumors with estrogen receptors (ER-positive) tend to respond better to hormonal treatments. ER-positive tumors are much more common in postmenopausal women.

Hormone receptors are determined from the biopsy specimen.

Other Factors

The biopsy also provides information about the tumor cells themselves—such as their type, growth rate, and grade—that influences the form and intensity of treatment offered.

Types of Treatment

After these factors are determined, the actual treatment plan is constructed. This centers around various combinations of four types of treatment:

- *Surgery:* physically removing as much of the tumor as possible in an operation
- *Radiation:* using high-dose X rays to kill cancer cells
- *Chemotherapy:* using drugs to kill cancer cells
- *Hormone therapy:* using hormones to stop the cancer cells from growing

---

Experimental Therapies

Newer forms of therapy are always being studied. Such experimental treatments include new anticancer drugs as well as gene therapy and biologic therapy, which uses the body's immune system to help fight cancer. Another is bone marrow transplantation, which involves the removal and replacement of blood-forming cells from the bone marrow. Experimental therapies are not widely available outside the major cancer centers, nor are they necessary for most women—most respond perfectly well to the standard therapies.

Which Treatment?

Today, unlike the 1950s, when radical mastectomy was the norm, doctors can draw on several decades of research and experience clearly showing that there are better ways of treating cancer than removing the entire breast. Treatments have been compared against one another in large numbers of women, and the standard treatments used today have emerged as the ones that help the most women.

Stage 0

Lobular carcinoma in situ (LCIS) is not really cancer but is a marker of increased risk for cancer. Some women receive no treat-

Should You Take Part in a Clinical Trial?
Progress in the fight against breast cancer depends on finding the most effective treatments, and the way to progress is by comparing newer promising treatments against standard, established treatments in highly controlled clinical studies. This is how better treatments will be found. It is a personal decision whether to participate. If you are interested, ask your doctor or call the National Cancer Institute (1-800-4-CANCER).

ment for LCIS but rather are followed closely with regular check-ups to determine whether actual breast cancer develops. In some cases, a controversial practice is to have surgery to remove both breasts (*prophylactic mastectomy*). A third, experimental approach for LCIS is to take *tamoxifen*. This anti-estrogen drug is being tested in a large number of women to determine whether breast cancer can be prevented from ever developing.

Ductal carcinoma in situ (DCIS) is the earliest form of breast cancer and, unlike LCIS, requires treatment. It is highly curable. The standard options consist of either limited surgery that removes only the cancer (*lumpectomy*) followed by *radiation therapy*, or surgery to remove the whole breast (*mastectomy*). Lumpectomy with and without hormonal therapy is being evaluated in research studies for its effectiveness.

Because DCIS and LCIS may be difficult to distinguish from each other but involve very different treatments, a second opinion may be a good idea before deciding about treatment in this stage.

Stage I and II

Stage I and II are both early breast cancers and highly treatable. These may be locally or regionally invasive forms of breast cancer, meaning the cancer has invaded the breast tissue outside the ducts or lobules but is still within the breast.

Treatment for these stages consists of surgery, but limited forms of breast removal may be possible. These include removal of only the cancer (*lumpectomy*) or a broader part of the breast (*partial* or *segmental* mastectomy), with both procedures followed by radiation therapy for four to six weeks. Some lymph nodes under the arm may also be removed to test for spread of cancer. Not all women may be appropriate candidates for lumpectomy because of the size or location of the tumor, multiple sites of tumors (multicentric disease), or for cosmetic considerations. The alternative approach is removal of the whole breast (*total* mastectomy), sometimes including the lining over the chest muscles (*modified radical* mastectomy) and some axillary lymph nodes.

These forms of surgery are followed by additional (*adjuvant*) chemotherapy and/or hormonal therapy, to prevent the cancer from recurring. For certain "good-risk" patients, no adjuvant therapy may be given.

Stage III

Women with Stage III breast cancer are divided into two groups. For those with Stage IIIA disease, which is considered operable, treatment plans often include surgery and radiation to remove or kill the tumor, followed by chemotherapy and/or hormonal therapy to stop the cancer from spreading. Surgery can be extensive, with either a modified radical or radical mastectomy, including some lymph nodes. Sometimes, chemotherapy may be given first, before surgery or radiation, to shrink the tumor. A lumpectomy may then be carried out.

When an advanced form of Stage III is present, termed Stage IIIB, radiation therapy may be given first to control the tumor, followed by chemotherapy or sometimes hormonal therapy to treat

---

Where to Get Treated, Locally or at a Cancer Center?
The National Cancer Institute (NCI) maintains a listing of more than fifty regional Cancer Centers that are involved in breast cancer research. These centers, which must pass a rigorous review by the NCI, offer the latest in treatments, both standard and experimental. Many local hospitals, while not involved in the experimental treatments, offer expert state-of-the-art care for breast and other cancers. The American Cancer Society or the NCI can recommend such qualified hospitals.

cancer that has spread. Surgery may be done later. Alternatively, chemotherapy may be given first, followed by surgery and/or radiation, which in turn is followed by more chemotherapy.

Newer therapies are being studied for this stage of disease, but they are not yet widely available. These include hormonal therapy, biologic agents, and high-dose chemotherapy with bone marrow transplantation.

Investigational Therapies

Information and up-to-date trial results concerning experimental treatments are available through the National Cancer Institute's Cancer Information Service—1-800-4-CANCER.

Stage IV

Treatment for Stage IV breast cancer usually consists of hormonal therapy or chemotherapy to control the spread of the cancer in distant parts of the body. Radiotherapy or mastectomy may be recommended to treat the local tumor, though not always. Radiation also may be used against the metastatic sites of cancer, depending on the effects of the tumor in those areas. Experimental therapies using new drugs and biologic therapies are also being evaluated.

It's Not Always Straightforward

Unfortunately, the criteria for treatment and the various forms of treatment themselves aren't perfect. The standard therapies, while helping most women, do not cure everyone. In some, the first treatment might not have a large enough effect, and another treatment has to be substituted. Other therapies that appear to bring about cures initially may be followed by a recurrence of cancer, or even a new cancer, in the following years.

In addition, side effects of treatment are somewhat unpredictable, and in an occasional woman, they may be so severe as to limit the amount of effective therapy that can be received. These side effects differ for each person, and they may even differ in the same person from one treatment to the next. Doctors try to plan treatments to strike a balance between the best chance of success versus the limitations of the treatments themselves.

Unproven Remedies?

When a cure is found for cancer, everyone will know. Many of the so-called "alternative" or unproven remedies, such as special diets or laughter, are okay to use as long as they don't prevent you from following the treatment your doctor prescribes, and as long as your doctor is aware of them.

Making a Decision

After all the discussion about stages and prognostic factors, if it sounds as though there still is some choice left in selecting treatments, you are right.

And who then makes the final decision? With the help of your doctor, *you do*.

Your doctor will recommend one treatment plan that probably is the best. He or she can explain those treatments and what the effects most likely will be. You should be sure to completely understand it and all its limitations and risks. Why was this treatment chosen? How successful is it expected to be? Are there alternatives?

Often, the decision revolves around tradeoffs between acceptable risk and more extensive treatment. For example, a woman with LCIS, or Stage 0 cancer, has to decide herself whether to forgo treatment in favor of regular checkups, or whether any risk, however slight, is too much risk.

The meeting with the doctor to discuss the treatment plan can be stressful. Because of the nature of the information being discussed, it may be difficult to listen to the options, ask the important questions, and then afterward remember all that's been said. Many women rely on a friend or family member to accompany them, who can ask additional questions, take notes, or be there for support. Writing down questions beforehand and taking notes during the meetings are other useful steps.

Before going ahead with any treatment, be sure that it is explained clearly and that you agree with that decision.

Your Treatment Team

Your primary physician may refer you to other specialists who will handle the different phases of your treatment. Your initial physician or any one of these specialist physicians may continue to work with you to coordinate your treatments and follow-up care. The specialists include:

- *Surgeon*—a doctor who performs surgery, such as biopsy and mastectomy

- *Plastic surgeon*—a doctor who specializes in rehabilitative and cosmetic surgery, including breast reconstruction

- *Pathologist*—a doctor who examines biopsy tissues under a microscope to see if cancer is present

- *Radiologist*—a doctor who uses X rays and other imaging methods, including mammography, to diagnose problems and diseases

- *Radiation oncologist*—a doctor who uses X rays to treat cancer

- *Radiation oncology nurse*—a nurse with special knowledge in radiation oncology, who will care for you during radiation therapy

- *Medical oncologist*—a doctor who administers anticancer drugs or chemotherapy

- *Nurse oncologist*—a nurse with special knowledge in medical oncology, who will care for you while chemotherapy is given

- *Physical therapist*—a specialist who helps in rehabilitation after surgery by using exercise, heat, and massage

It's Your Turn

1. What stage is your disease?
   ❑ 0*   ❑ I   ❑ II (A or B?)
   ❑ III (A or B?)   ❑ IV
   *If Stage 0, is it DCIS or LCIS?_____

2. Are the lymph nodes involved?
   ❑ Yes (node-positive)
   ❑ No (node-negative)

3. Do you have any poor prognostic (risk) factors?
How aggressive is the tumor?

_____

_____

_____

4. What treatment plan has been recommended for you?
   ❑ Surgery. What kind? _____
   ❑ Radiation therapy
   ❑ Chemotherapy
   ❑ Hormone therapy
   ❑ Other. What kind? _____

5. Do you understand why these treatments are being recommended?
   ❑ Yes
   ❑ No*
*Talk to your doctor to get a clearer explanation.

6. Do you understand the treatment's risks or drawbacks?
   ❑ Yes
   ❑ No*
*Talk to your doctor to get a clearer explanation.

7. Do you agree with the treatment plan proposed for you?
   ❑ Yes
   ❑ No*
*Talk to your doctor to get a clearer explanation.

4

Surgery

FOR MOST WOMEN with breast cancer, surgery is the first step in treatment. Over the past several decades and through many clinical trials, mastectomy (removing the entire breast) has proven to be one effective way to treat breast cancer and prevent its recurrence. But losing a breast, even when this entails curing breast cancer, can carry great emotional as well as physical trauma.

However, thanks to newer forms of surgery, mastectomy is now only *one* of several options. In more than half of women with breast cancer, a less extreme, breast-conserving procedure may be possible—without sacrificing the chance of success. In fact, since 1990, the National Cancer Institute has recommended that breast-conserving surgery is the preferable form of therapy for all women with early-stage breast cancer.

As we discussed in the last chapter, the type of surgery recommended by your physician depends on various factors—the size of the tumor, its type, whether the cancer has spread, your medical history, age, and some other factors. But several different kinds of surgery may be effective, and *your feelings may be the ultimate deciding factor.*

Margins of Safety I

The goal of all surgery, whether a mastectomy or breast-conserving surgery, is to remove the entire tumor while saving as much of the breast as possible. To do this, the surgeon must remove some normal breast tissue surrounding the tumor. This rim of normal tissue, called a "margin" on the laboratory report, is generally at least half an inch (one cm) wide all around the tumor.

For small tumors, the amount of tissue taken may hardly be noticeable. For larger tumors or those that have spread, more breast tissue is removed. The ducts around some tumors also may have cancer cells in them, a condition termed EIC, or *extensive intravascular component*. This tissue also needs to be removed and may result in a larger surgery, depending on its extent. Thus, the amount of breast tissue removed varies greatly.

Margins of Safety II

Surgery alone is usually not enough to be certain the cancer is cured. Microscopic groups of cancer cells can escape detection in the breast during surgery. Other cells might have already escaped from the breast into the rest of the body (metastasis). To prevent these cells from growing into a new tumor, other forms of therapy are given after surgery. For this reason, the more limited surgeries, like lumpectomy, are usually followed by radiation. If the surgery shows that cells are likely to have metastasized, chemotherapy and/or hormonal therapy will be needed.

Breast-conserving Surgeries

In contrast to mastectomy, in which the breast is removed entirely, breast-conserving surgery removes only a small part, leaving most of the normal breast intact, as well as sensation to the breast.

Since the 1970s and 1980s, clinical studies have shown that breast-conserving surgery, when combined with radiation, provides equal results in terms of survival after breast cancer, compared to mastectomy. For this reason, the more limited surgery is preferred by most women, because it allows them to keep their breast and has better cosmetic results.

There are two basic types of breast-conserving surgery: lumpectomy and partial (or segmental) mastectomy.

Lumpectomy

Lumpectomy is usually an outpatient procedure that involves removing only the breast lump through a small incision, plus a small

rim (the "margin") of normal breast tissue around it. Through a separate incision, some lymph nodes are also removed from under the arm to check for spread of the cancer outside the breast. Often, a lumpectomy is simply a one-step procedure given as part of the initial biopsy, *with radiation treatment following it.*

Lumpectomy is also referred to as tylectomy, wide excision, and tumorectomy.

Since 1990, lumpectomy has been the recommended form of surgery for women with early-stage breast cancer. It is preferable because it preserves almost all of the normal breast, leaving its normal sensation intact. The resulting scar is small, and there is little change in breast size or shape. Other problems that accompany major surgery—general anesthesia, infection, muscle weakness, and lymphedema (swelling of the arm)—are also largely avoided.

Although lumpectomy can be used to remove tumors up to about two inches, the procedure is not for everyone. Women with larger tumors, especially if they have small breasts, may find the final appearance unacceptable. In these cases, mastectomy with breast reconstruction may provide better cosmetic results. Other reasons that lumpectomy might not be a good option include:

- Multiple tumors (so-called multicentric disease)

- Widespread flecks of calcium (microcalcifications) found on the mammogram, which suggest diffuse spread of the cancer within the breast

- Tumor located under the nipple, which may lead to a poor cosmetic result

- Young age (under thirty-five to forty years)

- Presence of an unrelated condition called collagen vascular disease (lupus, scleroderma, etc.)

Despite the procedure's relative ease of performance and better cosmetic results, lumpectomy should not be regarded as a "less aggressive" form of therapy. Nor is it necessarily better tolerated by the patient, over the short term, than mastectomy. In fact, the radiation treatments that follow are lengthy, involving daily treatments for up to six weeks. Furthermore, because cancer may recur in the treated breast, long-term, regular breast checkups are necessary.

As you can see, though lumpectomy followed by radiation is a milestone improvement in the treatment of breast cancer, for numerous reasons mastectomy may remain the best option for many women.

Partial Mastectomy

One step beyond lumpectomy is the partial mastectomy, in which a bit more breast tissue is removed. This is also performed as an outpatient procedure and likewise is intended for small, Stage I or II tumors, under two inches in size.

Partial mastectomy removes up to a quarter of the breast tissue, including the tumor and a wedge of surrounding normal breast tissue. Some lymph nodes under the arm will also be excised, and a portion of the lining of the underlying chest muscle may be removed. Radiation therapy always follows partial mastectomy.

As with lumpectomy, partial mastectomy spares most of the breast, preserving its size, shape, and sensation, though not quite as well as lumpectomy. If the breasts are small or medium in size, there may result a noticeable change in the breast's shape or size compared to the other breast. Also, because the procedure is somewhat more extensive than lumpectomy, there is a greater possibility of arm swelling (lymphedema).

Partial mastectomy is also referred to as segmental mastectomy or quadrantectomy.

The radiation therapy that is administered after both lumpectomy and partial mastectomy brings its own set of possible problems (see Chapter 5).

Mastectomy

Despite the advantages of breast-conserving therapy, many women choose the option of complete breast removal—a mastectomy. For some other women, because of their tumor's location or the extent of disease, it is the treatment of choice.

Modified Radical Mastectomy

Modified radical mastectomy is also termed "total mastectomy with axillary lymph node dissection."

The modified radical mastectomy is the most common form of breast cancer surgery today. It became the standard form of breast cancer surgery in the 1970s, when it was discovered that survival rates of modified radical mastectomy were equal to those of radical mastectomy, but with better cosmetic results and fewer complications.

In the modified radical mastectomy, the entire breast is removed, along with the underarm lymph nodes and the lining over the chest muscles. If the tumor is deep in the breast, one of the underlying chest muscles is sometimes removed. Radiation therapy is usually not given after this surgery.

The advantages of mastectomy are that it removes all of the tumor confined to the breast, avoids the follow-up radiation treatments, and, by removing all the breast, greatly reduces the chance of cancer recurrence in that breast. But it will not prevent cancer from developing elsewhere if cancer cells have already invaded adjacent tissue or metastasized, which often occurs. In these instances, additional cancer therapy is needed.

The disadvantage of this form of mastectomy is that it leaves a long scar and no breast, although breast reconstruction can be performed after it. The modified surgery is preferred to the older radical mastectomy because the chest muscles remain intact, preserving arm strength and giving a more natural appearance to the upper chest under the collarbone. Arm swelling (lymphedema) may occur, but is less likely and less severe than with radical mastectomy.

Radical Mastectomy

For most of this century (until the early 1970s), radical mastectomy was the standard operation for all breast cancer. This surgery consists of removing the entire breast, the chest muscles under the breast, all of the underarm lymph nodes, and some fat and skin around the breast. This surgery is now employed only for women who have very extensive tumors and is rarely used today.

The surgery leaves a long scar and a large depression on the chest extending from beneath the collarbone. It may also cause swelling of the arm (lymphedema), some loss of muscle power in the arm, restricted shoulder motion, and arm numbness and discomfort. Breast reconstruction is more difficult than with the less extensive modified radical mastectomy.

The Halsted Radical Mastectomy

Radical mastectomy, also termed the Halsted radical mastectomy, was developed in the late 1800s and named after the famous U.S. surgeon William S. Halsted. As he envisioned it, cancer spread in a straight line from the breast to other areas, and so he devised a surgical procedure that eliminated the tumor, plus the areas where it might spread. The surgery was extensive, but it was much more successful than anything else done at the time.

In fairness to Dr. Halsted, cancer in the late 1800s was often detected at a much later stage than it is today. His surgery offered such improvement over the other existing techniques that it soon was adopted as the standard treatment for breast cancer, and it remained the main form of treatment for the next seventy years.

Total Mastectomy

Total mastectomy is a limited version of the modified radical mastectomy. This procedure removes only the breast. A few of the underarm lymph nodes closest to the breast also are excised to check whether cancer has spread there. Unlike the other forms of mastectomy, total mastectomy may be followed by radiation therapy.

This surgery is seldom used, in general mainly for women with very small, noninvasive tumors considered to have little chance of spread beyond the breast. It is also used for women who want breast removal to prevent cancer (prophylactic mastectomy). Breast reconstruction can follow.

Total mastectomy is also termed simple mastectomy.

Lymph Nodes

In all types of breast cancer surgery, the surgeon removes some lymph nodes from under the arm. A small group of these, about five to ten, might be removed in a lumpectomy, or many more in a modified radical mastectomy, depending on whether the cancer is believed to have spread. These lymph nodes are sent to the pathologist, who examines them under the microscope to see whether they have been invaded by cancer.

The number of lymph nodes containing cancer cells is used to estimate the likelihood that the cancer has spread to other organs (metastasized). If no lymph nodes are involved (*node-negative*), the cancer is more likely to be confined to the breast, and local treatment of the breast with radiotherapy may be the only other treatment needed after surgery. If any nodes are involved (*node-positive*), then it is assumed that the cancer has spread farther, meaning that systemic chemotherapy and/or hormonal treatment will be needed.

Removing lymph nodes is not entirely harmless. It can cause swelling of the arm, called *lymphedema*, especially if many are removed, as is the case in mastectomies.

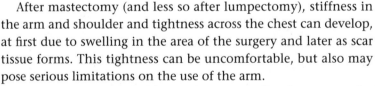

How Many Lymph Nodes to Sample?

The number of lymph nodes taken varies widely among women, and the surgeon does not set out to remove any specific number. The lymph nodes are encased in a layer of fat, making it impossible to tell how many are present when a sample is removed. So some patients may have only a few nodes removed, and another patient may have dozens taken out. Despite how many are removed, it is the number of nodes containing cancer that indicates whether the cancer has spread.

Postsurgical Exercises

After mastectomy (and less so after lumpectomy), stiffness in the arm and shoulder and tightness across the chest can develop, at first due to swelling in the area of the surgery and later as scar tissue forms. This tightness can be uncomfortable, but also may pose serious limitations on the use of the arm.

To help reduce this problem, a day or two after the surgery, the surgeon or a physical therapist will demonstrate some simple arm exercises designed to relax the muscles and promote joint movement. These exercises, called *range-of-motion exercises,* are just a series of ordinary arm movements—moving the arm back and forth and in circles, or clenching the hand into a fist and then relaxing it (more about these in Chapter 8).

Despite any pain initially, it is important that the exercises are done as prescribed. Otherwise, the stiffness worsens. The exercises also may help prevent lymphedema, which is the swelling in the arm that can occur after surgery.

Breast Reconstruction

Following a mastectomy, many women may be satisfied to wear an artificial breast form (prosthesis) that fits inside the bra. Others, however, may want to consider a surgical breast reconstruction, which may be performed at the same time as the mastectomy.

Several techniques can be used to recreate the shape of the natural breast, all with very good cosmetic results. A surgeon may insert a silicone gel or saline-filled implant under the skin or use body tissue taken from another site on the woman's body.

Silicone and Saline Implants

The most frequent and simplest type of breast reconstruction involves an implant, a balloonlike device filled with silicone gel or saline (salt water), which is inserted beneath the skin or muscle of the chest. Sometimes an expander, which is a partially filled implant, is used to stretch the skin first. The surgeon then injects additional fluid into the expander a few times over several weeks until the final size is reached.

Over recent years, some women have reported problems following silicone implants, including cancer, arthritis, and skin rashes. However, research so far has not proven that these problems are related to the implants, and silicone implants are considered relatively safe. However, because questions about safety continue to arise, silicone implants are available only to women having mastectomies who are willing to participate in clinical research trials.

Saline-filled implants have not been associated with these problems.

Muscle Flap Procedures

As an alternative to the artificial implants, natural tissue (including muscle, skin, and fat) can be removed from other body sites and transferred to the chest to recreate a natural breast mound.

In the *latissimus dorsi flap procedure*, a flap of muscle and skin is transferred from the back and folded around under the skin to the front of the chest. This creates a pocket into which a silicone or saline implant is placed.

The *transverse rectus abdominis muscle* (TRAM) flap uses extra tissue and muscle from the lower abdomen. The muscle is cut from the lower abdomen and folded back under the skin to create a breast mound. Skin taken from the lower stomach is then grafted over the new breast.

Another procedure uses a *free flap* consisting of extra skin, fat, and muscle taken from the buttocks, thigh, or abdomen. This is a more complicated and time-consuming procedure that involves sewing the blood vessels together to restore a blood supply to the flap where it is placed on the chest. It is reserved for women who cannot have the other flap procedures.

For all of the reconstruction procedures, a nipple and areola are made from skin taken from other areas. Because of the questions about silicone, the TRAM procedure has gained wider use in recent years. The use of implants, however, still remains the most widely used technique.

Reach to Recovery

Following a mastectomy, a woman may feel emotionally upset or depressed about loss of the breast. There are also the practical matters of finding a bra that fits (even if breast reconstruction is done immediately) or selecting a breast prosthesis to fit into the bra. A volunteer from Reach to Recovery, which is a program of the American Cancer Society composed of women who have had breast cancer, can talk with you and help ease the problems encountered during this time. Contact your local ACS branch for information.

Cancer Recurrence

Cancer may recur in a small percentage of women having breast-conserving surgery (lumpectomy). This usually occurs in the same breast, usually within the first three to five years after surgery, and often in the same area as the first tumor. The treatment in these cases is mastectomy. The outcome for these women is the same as if they had had the mastectomy initially, so a lumpectomy is not "riskier" or less adequate than mastectomy.

Local recurrence of cancer—in the same breast—is uncommon after mastectomy, but it can occur if any cancer cells remain, either in the remaining breast tissue or in the muscle underlying the breast. More likely, the cancer may return as a metastasis affecting another site. The chances of metastasis increase with the advancing stages of cancer.

For all women, the opposite healthy breast, too, should be checked regularly for lumps and with annual mammograms.

Planning Ahead

When a woman is first faced with breast cancer, her primary concern is getting rid of the cancer. Somehow, it may seem unimportant or even vain to think about "plastic surgery." But if you feel that at some future point you might want to consider a breast reconstruction, this should be discussed with your surgeon before the mastectomy. The procedure may be done later, but the position of the incision can affect the reconstruction process. The reconstructed breasts do not interfere with other cancer treatments that may be needed or with detecting breast cancer recurrence.

Lymphedema and Other Complications

As with any surgery, a variety of complications can occur. Some of these, such as infection or hematoma (a leak of blood that forms a lump or bruiselike spot), are acute or short-term problems. They tend to be rare, occur soon after the surgery, and usually resolve on their own. Some complications, however, tend to be more persistent.

Lymphedema is swelling of the arm on the side of the mastectomy. This swelling occurs when the lymph nodes under the arm are removed, so that the lymph fluid in the arm cannot drain. Infection of the arm occurs more readily, which in turn can cause more swelling. Simple scratches or burns, or even wearing jewelry, might also incite this swelling. Your doctor will explain arm exercises that can help prevent this problem (see Chapter 8).

Lymphedema was more common in the past, when the more extensive radical mastectomy was frequently performed, but it still tends to occur whenever lymph nodes are removed. It is uncommon after the more limited breast-conserving surgeries. But lymphedema is a lifelong problem and can be difficult to resolve once it starts.

Numbness of the arm or chest area can occur if the nerve passing through the underarm region is injured during surgery. The inside of the upper arm will be numb, but full feeling usually returns slowly within a year.

Back pain may be experienced because the removal of one breast can cause an imbalance in posture. This can be corrected by using a heavier breast form (prosthesis) or with breast reconstruction.

It's Your Turn

1. What type of surgery has been recommended or performed in your case?
- ❏ Lumpectomy
- ❏ Partial mastectomy (quadrantectomy, segmental mastectomy)
- ❏ Modified radical mastectomy
- ❏ Other: _____

2. Is breast-conserving surgery (lumpectomy or partial mastectomy) an option for you? If not, why?

_____

_____

3. What additional cancer treatments will be needed after surgery?
- ❏ None
- ❏ Chemotherapy
- ❏ Radiation therapy
- ❏ Hormone therapy
- ❏ Other: _____

4. Has the doctor recommended any postsurgical exercises?
- ❏ Yes   ❏ No

5. If lymph nodes were removed during surgery, did any show cancer?

❏ None   ❏ Less than 4   ❏ More than 4

6. If you are having a mastectomy, will breast reconstruction be done? When?

❏ Yes, at the time of surgery
❏ I don't know*
❏ Yes, at a later date*
❏ Not interested

*If you think you might want to have breast reconstruction at a later time or aren't sure, discuss this with your surgeon. The surgical incisions may be placed to allow the later reconstruction.

5

Radiation Therapy

SINCE 1990, THE National Cancer Institute has recommended that all women with early-stage breast cancer be treated with breast-conserving therapy. This approach involves surgery as the first step, followed by radiation. Used in combination, lumpectomy and radiation provide cure rates that are equal to those of mastectomy.

As more women opt for this breast-conserving therapy, the use of radiation therapy has been rising over the past decade. In addition, radiation therapy has other roles in the treatment of breast cancer.

What Is Radiation?

Radiation is an invisible form of energy that can penetrate the body's soft tissues (skin, muscle, and fat). In a low-level form, this energy is used to make images, such as chest X rays or mammograms. When this energy is increased 500 to 1000 times and beamed into a small area, radiation gains the power to destroy cancer.

Radiation kills cancer cells by damaging their DNA, making it irreparable and causing the cells to stop functioning and die. Normal, healthy cells getting in the way of the radiation beam also will be damaged, but fortunately they can recover.

Why Is It Used?

Most often, radiation therapy, also called *radiotherapy*, is given after breast-conserving surgery for breast cancer.

The goal of breast surgery, no matter how limited or extensive the procedure, is to remove all cancer from the breast. But microscopic groups of cancer cells that have spread from the original tumor can be left behind. Despite the surgeon's thoroughness, these cells cannot be seen or detected at the time of surgery, and within a few years, any cells left behind can grow into a new tumor.

This is why radiation is so important after surgery—to kill off those remaining, "hidden" cancer cells.

At other times, radiation therapy is given to shrink the tumor or control its spread. Shrinking the tumor may make it easier for other therapies, such as surgery or chemotherapy, to remove or destroy the remaining tumor. Shrinking a tumor is also a way to relieve symptoms caused by the tumor's pressure on neighboring normal tissues, such as in metastatic disease.

Is Lumpectomy Alone Good Enough?

For very small tumors, doctors tested whether lumpectomy by itself, without radiation, would be enough to cure breast cancer. In older research studies, cancer recurred within a few years in many women who had lumpectomy alone, often in the very same area as the previous tumor. These tumors were caused by the cancer cells missed by surgery. In contrast, when radiation was given after lumpectomy, it prevented cancer recurrence in most of these women. And in those women who had a recurrence, mastectomy could still be performed, with the final result being just as life-saving as if a mastectomy had been done in the first place. But not to be forgotten is that most women are able to keep their breast by having a lumpectomy followed by radiation.

Who Should Have Radiotherapy?

Radiation therapy is generally used in three situations when treating breast cancer:

Breast-conserving Surgery

After lumpectomy or partial mastectomy in Stage 0, I, and II cancers, radiation is used to kill any remaining cancer cells and thereby prevent cancer recurrence. It is given to all of the remaining breast and also to the underarm lymph nodes on the treated side if cancer was detected within those nodes.

Breast-conserving surgery is always used with radiotherapy because there is a high likelihood of cancer recurrence in the breast if radiotherapy is omitted.

In some women with early-stage breast cancer, chemotherapy may be given *before* radiation treatments. Some research has shown a benefit to this sequence of treatments in women with

Stage II cancer at high risk for metastases, but additional research into this approach is underway.

Radiation is usually not given after a mastectomy because the mastectomy removes all breast tissue and presumably all cancer cells in that area as well. However, in a few situations, radiation may be indicated. For example, if during a mastectomy, the cancer is found to lie deep in the breast, perhaps involving the chest muscles, radiotherapy may be given. Likewise, radiotherapy may be used to treat a recurrence of tumor within the chest muscle following a mastectomy.

Advanced Cancers

In later-stage cancers (Stage III or IV), radiation may be given before or after chemotherapy and surgery to stop tumor growth or to shrink the tumor. As the cancer shrinks following radiation treatment, its borders become more distinct, making the tumor easier for the surgeon to remove.

Women with Stage III cancer or with inflammatory breast cancer may be treated with radiation after first receiving chemotherapy. Here, the radiation is intended to control the tumor locally in the breast. This is followed by surgery and more chemotherapy.

Metastatic Cancers

In metastatic cancer, radiation may be given to other parts of the body in order to shrink tumors occurring outside the breast. This may help to relieve symptoms, such as bone pain, and is termed *palliative* (to make less severe).

Who Should *Not* Have Radiotherapy?

A few people have medical conditions that prohibit the use of radiation treatment. These include:

- *Prior history of radiation to the chest area:* Women treated previously for an earlier episode of breast cancer or for another condition, such as Hodgkin's disease, cannot have more radiation to the same area. However, radiation administered elsewhere to the body in the past, even to the other breast, does not prohibit breast irradiation.

- *Pregnancy:* Radiotherapy may have harmful effects on the developing fetus.
- *Scleroderma or lupus erythematosus:* These uncommon diseases can precipitate excessive reactions in the blood vessels and skin exposed to radiation. (For this reason, persons with these diseases should even avoid sunlight because of its low-level radiation.)

In some situations, radiotherapy may not be medically effective. Some of these reasons are the same ones for avoiding lumpectomy, such as:

- Multiple tumors in the same breast
- When small calcium specks appear widespread on the mammogram, meaning the cancer itself is too widespread to be treated with lumpectomy and radiation

Finally, radiation may cause excessive distortion of the breast's shape or skin thickening, producing a cosmetically unacceptable result in some cases. Although the treatment would cure the cancer, the woman might choose to have mastectomy followed by breast reconstruction in the cases of:

- Large, pendulous breasts
- Small breasts containing a silicone or saline implant (implants may be placed after radiotherapy has ended)
- Older women (it may cause considerable breast shrinkage and thickening)

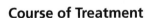

Course of Treatment

In breast-conserving therapy, radiation treatment begins about two weeks after surgery or as soon as the skin heals from the inci-

Helpful Exercises

Things you can do after surgery to help regain full motion of your arm in preparation for radiotherapy are explained in Chapter 8, under "Arm Exercises." Your doctor or nurse will explain when to start and which exercises are best for you.

sion. Also, by this time, the woman should be able to raise her arm over her head without much pain. This position is typically used while treatment is given.

Radiation treatment is overseen by a *radiation oncologist*, a doctor specializing in the treatment of cancer by X rays. A *radiation therapist* is the person who actually sets up the treatments each day and operates the equipment. Treatment is generally given in the radiation therapy or radiology department of a hospital.

Treatment Planning

The first appointment with the radiation oncologist is for a planning session, called a *simulation*. During this visit, various X rays and mammograms are taken to plot the location of the tumor site in the breast and the positions of the ribs, lungs, and heart. Usually, the radiation beam is angled to enter the side of the breast, aimed away from the rest of the body, so that underlying organs are minimally affected.

At the simulation, the radiation therapist outlines the site to be treated, called the *treatment port*, with a series of tiny dots or lines marked on and around the breast. You should be careful not to wash off these marks, since this is how the therapist knows where to direct the treatment on later visits.

A centigray (cGy) is the unit used by radiologists to measure doses of radiation. A regular chest X ray uses less than 1 cGy.

Calculating the Dose

During the simulation, a doctor called a *dosimetrist* calculates the total dose of radiation required, based on the size of the tumor removed and its depth in the breast. This dose is broken down into daily treatments calculated to cause the most damage to cancer cells and the least damage to normal cells.

Typically, 4500 to 5000 cGy of radiation is given for breast cancer. The dose is delivered at about 180 to 200 cGy per day for five days a week, for five to six weeks.

Treatment Sessions

During the treatment sessions, you lie on a table, very still, with your arm over your head. The radiation machine is mounted on an arm over the table and moves during treatment to deliver the radiation from several angles. The machine's movement is controlled by the radiation therapist, who watches via a video monitor in the next room.

Each therapy session lasts about half an hour, although radiation is given only for about one to two minutes of that time. You cannot feel or hear the radiation, and it does not hurt.

A *radiation oncology nurse* will be available to answer questions and to help care for you during this time.

The Booster Dose

After the first series of radiation treatments is finished, an extra "boost" of radiation is frequently given to the site where the tumor was removed. Cancers often recur in this area, so the boost delivers a concentrated dose of radiation, about 1000 to 1500 cGy, to ensure any "hidden" cancer cells are destroyed.

Booster treatments can be delivered by two methods. One way is with an external "electron" beam machine similar to the machine used for the regular radiotherapy. These treatments are much like the other sessions and last for about two weeks.

A second method, called *brachytherapy,* involves implanting several small plastic tubes directly into the tumor site in the breast. Inside these tubes are tiny radioactive pellets that give off radiation in the region of the removed tumor. The tubes are left in place for a day or two and are removed under local anesthetic, just as sutures or stitches are removed. During this time, you need to be hospitalized. Visitors are allowed only for about an hour a day, to prevent harmful exposure to low-level radiation that might escape.

Side Effects

Most people receiving radiation therapy will have only mild side effects, or none at all. For some people, though, the side effects can be significant, and for these few, it is not unusual to stop treatment for a week or so to allow them to subside.

The side effects may start after about two weeks of treatment and disappear within a few weeks after treatment is finished. The nurse or doctor will help manage any side effects, which include:

Fatigue

Many people having radiotherapy feel fatigued. It results from the effects of radiation on normal cells, stress related to the cancer, and the daily trips for treatment. It disappears within a few weeks after treatment is finished, but until then, it is best for activities to be limited.

Skin Problems

Redness, irritation, and dryness of the skin are common after radiation. Usually, a sunburnlike redness develops over the breast, which ultimately peels, just like a sunburn. This may progress to irritation and tanning, and it gradually fades after treatment ends. The doctor or nurse can recommend ways to relieve any itching or discomfort; it is important not to use any home remedies or other skin products (powders, creams, deodorants, oils) during this time, as these can interfere with the radiation treatment.

A few women develop a "moist" reaction, which is wetness, particularly in skin folds around the breast. These areas can become very sore. Others experience "dry" reactions in which the skin becomes very dry, cracked, and irritated. Again, the doctor or nurse can advise how to relieve these problems.

How Will It Look?

The advantages of breast-conserving therapy are preservation of the breast and a better cosmetic appearance of the breast afterward. Under the best circumstances, the treated breast feels and looks very similar to the normal breast.

However, radiotherapy can cause some temporary skin changes on the breast. Some women have small light or dark spots that persist after treatment or hardening or stiffening of skin around the treatment site. Rarely, there may be loss of sensation in the breast, breast shrinkage, or distortion of the breast's shape.

Swelling

Some slight breast swelling, often with tenderness, is common during treatment. This swelling disappears gradually over a year, and afterward, the breast may shrink and feel thicker or firmer (called *induration* or *fibrosis*).

Because the radiation field is limited to the breast, other common side effects of radiation such as hair loss, nausea and vomiting, and loss of appetite do not occur. If the lymph nodes in the neck are treated, there sometimes may be dryness of the mouth or difficulty in swallowing.

Complications

Fewer than 5 percent of women experience any long-term complications after radiotherapy, thanks to marked improvements in radiation techniques and equipment in recent years. A few problems may still occur, however, including:

Rib Fractures: Some radiation to the breast may reach the ribs, causing the bone to become thin. As a result, minor trauma to the chest (for instance, from a fall or minor car accident) or even sneezing may cause a rib fracture. Such a fracture may or may not be painful.

Lymphedema: Just as with surgery, swelling of the arm may occur if the lymph nodes under the arm are included in the radiation field. Surgery to remove lymph nodes makes lymphedema likely, and subsequent radiotherapy to the underarm lymph nodes increases its occurrence by causing the lymph vessels to contract.

Nerve Damage: If the underarm lymph nodes are treated with radiation, on rare occasions the nerve running through that region to the arm may be affected. This causes a tingling sensation or weakness in the arm or hand.

Pneumonitis: After the radiation treatment is finished and for up to three to six months afterward, some women may notice a flulike illness with a cough. This occurs because the radiation causes part of the lung to become inflamed. It often goes away without treatment, though some doctors may prescribe corticosteroid-type medications. A small patch of lung scarring might be seen on subsequent X rays.

Pericarditis: Inflammation of the lining of the heart was seen more often in the past than today. It occurs when the left breast, which lies over the heart, is irradiated. Fever and chest pain with breathing are the main symptoms of pericarditis.

Second Cancers: Today's lower doses of radiation rarely cause secondary tumors, and any cancer developing in subsequent years is probably not caused by the radiation. The cancers seen have included sarcomas and leukemia. There is some question whether radiotherapy might cause cancer in the opposite, untreated breast, particularly in younger women; proper shielding of the opposite breast during radiation treatments is designed to help avoid this risk.

Because the side effects and complications may be more severe in women who simultaneously receive radiation and chemotherapy, these treatments are generally planned so that they do not overlap. In many cases, radiation is begun a few weeks after the completion of chemotherapy treatments.

Fertility

Although radiotherapy is not given during pregnancy, it will not affect a woman's ability to become pregnant later. Also, it does not affect the ovaries and causes no menstruation problems or birth defects. Successful breast-feeding with the treated breast has been reported in a few women, but it usually isn't possible. But the ability to breast-feed with the other breast is preserved.

Coping

People have different reactions to radiation therapy. Although it is possible to maintain normal routines, adjustments in daily life should be made for the fatigue and other side effects. Fewer activities than usual help preserve strength for the task at hand. Family, friends, and coworkers should be asked to lend assistance for a while. This isn't a sign of weakness, just common sense.

Treatment sessions usually will be scheduled at the same time each day, although these can be moved if problems arise. The staff at the treatment center can recommend ways to relieve side effects, will watch for other problems, and can answer questions. These regular appointments also offer a chance to meet and talk with other women having the same treatments.

Remember, radiation treatment does not make you radioactive, so don't worry about hugging children, grandchildren, or loved ones. After all, hugs are good medicine, too. Some other guidelines to remember are:

1. Get plenty of rest. Expect to sleep longer than usual.

2. Eat a balanced, healthy diet to help prevent weight loss and further fatigue.

3. Avoid tight clothing in the treatment area. Wearing loose cotton clothes or going braless can help.

4. Wash the area with lukewarm water.

5. Avoid using soaps, lotions, deodorants, perfumes, powders, or other substances in the treated area, except those approved by your doctor. These may irritate the skin or even interfere with treatment.

6. Do not apply heat (e.g., a heating pad) or cold (e.g., an ice pack) to the area.

7. Avoid shaving the underarm on the treated side. Use an electric shaver if you must.

8. Protect the breast area from the sun. Continue to protect the skin and use sunscreen freely for at least the first year after treatment has ended.

If you have questions, your doctor, nurse, and radiation therapist are the best people to ask. They can advise you about your treatment and side effects, any medicines you might need to take, or other medical concerns you may have.

It's Your Turn

1. Why is the doctor recommending radiation treatments for your breast cancer?
   - ❏ Following surgery, as part of breast-conserving therapy
   - ❏ To shrink the tumor before removing it surgically
   - ❏ To treat a recurrence after mastectomy

2. Have you previously had radiotherapy to the breast or chest region?
   - ❏ Yes*   ❏ No

*If yes, be sure your doctor is aware of the fact.

3. Do you have any conditions that might prohibit the use of radiation therapy or limit its effectiveness?*
   - ❏ Pregnancy
   - ❏ Collagen vascular disease (scleroderma, lupus)
   - ❏ Other

*If so, discuss these with your doctor before starting treatment.

4. Are you having any side effects from the radiation?

_____

_____

5. Are you:
   - ❏ Getting plenty of rest?
   - ❏ Eating a balanced diet?
   - ❏ Avoiding tight clothing in the treatment area?
   - ❏ Washing the area with lukewarm water?
   - ❏ Using only skin creams or lotions approved by your doctor?

6

Chemotherapy

FOLLOWING TREATMENT with surgery and radiation, some undetectable cancer cells may remain. These cells can be hidden in the
breast or, more likely, they may have spread outside the breast into
other parts of the body. Over time, these cells can multiply and
reappear in the form of new tumor sites.

To "clean up" these leftover cancer cells and prevent a recurrence of the cancer, additional treatment, called *adjuvant therapy*,
is needed after the surgery or radiation.

Until recently, adjuvant treatments were given only to women
whose breast cancer was known to have spread from the breast. It
was routinely included in the treatment plan for advanced Stage III
or IV cancers and for recurrent cancer. But today adjuvant treatments
are given to many women with early-stage breast cancer, meaning
most women are now possible candidates for adjuvant therapy.

An Overview of Adjuvant Therapy

Adjuvant means "in addition to," and in cancer therapy it refers
to treatments used in addition to the primary treatments of
surgery and radiation.

Chemotherapy and hormonal therapy are the two main adjuvant treatments for breast cancer. *Chemotherapy* uses anticancer
drugs to destroy the cancer cells. *Hormonal therapies* consist of
drugs that block the cancer cells from using estrogen, one of the
body's natural hormones, to help them grow faster.

Chemotherapy and hormonal therapy are given for the same
purpose: to kill the cancer cells that are outside the breast. Each is
used in certain situations and sometimes may be given together.
Hormonal therapy is discussed more fully in the next chapter,
but some of what we say here about the uses of chemotherapy also
applies to hormonal therapy.

Local or Systemic?

The adjuvant therapies—chemotherapy and hormonal therapy—are *systemic*,
which means that the drugs enter the bloodstream and travel through the
entire body, killing cancer cells wherever they are found. Surgery and radiation,
in contrast, are *local* therapies. They have their effect on cancer cells in only one
area of the body—the breast—or in specific metastatic sites.

Who Gets Adjuvant Therapy?

To decide who needs systemic adjuvant treatment, doctors first look at the lymph nodes. (As you recall from Chapter 4, some lymph nodes are removed during surgery and sent to the pathologist for examination.) Other indications include metastatic and recurrent cancers.

Lymph Node–Positive

If the lymph nodes show evidence of cancer cells in them (node-positive), then there is a chance the breast cancer has gained access to the rest of the body. Women with this condition traditionally have been offered adjuvant therapy, with chemotherapy, hormonal therapy, or sometimes both.

Lymph Node–Negative

Until the mid-1980s, women with early Stage I or II cancers received no additional treatment beyond the initial surgery and radiation. Most did not have cancer in their lymph nodes (node-negative), and they were considered low risk for more cancer. But cancer recurred in about 20 to 30 percent of these women nevertheless.

To explain these recurrences, the experts now believe that breast cancer spreads to the rest of the body much earlier than was previously thought.

And so these women too, except for those with the earliest and smallest tumors (less than half an inch), may benefit from adjuvant therapy following surgery and radiation.

Metastatic Cancer

If the cancer has spread to other organs of the body, chemotherapy or hormonal therapy, and sometimes both, becomes the primary treatment to control the cancer.

Recurrent Cancer

If breast cancer recurs, surgery and/or radiation therapy is used if the second tumor is confined to the breast. But hormones, chemotherapy, or both may be added to reduce the chances that the cancer will recur again.

By these guidelines, a large number of women might need some form of adjuvant therapy. To decide which form—chemotherapy or hormonal, or both—doctors rely on several signs, but more on these later. First, an introduction to chemotherapy.

The Purpose of Chemotherapy

Chemotherapy is the use of anticancer drugs given to kill cancer cells that may have escaped surgery or radiation and spread to other parts of the body. It is a form of *systemic therapy*, meaning it works throughout the body, destroying cancer cells wherever they exist, from the skin to the bones and all parts in between.

In addition to killing the cancer, chemotherapy sometimes is used to shrink a tumor, which then makes it easier for surgery or radiation therapy to remove or destroy. Shrinking a tumor can also reduce the symptoms it is causing, such as bone pain. This use is termed *palliative,* meaning "to make less severe."

How Chemotherapy Works

Anticancer drugs attack rapidly dividing cells, which are typical of cancer. At particular points in the tumor cell's life cycle, certain drugs interfere with enzymes produced by the tumor cell that help it grow. Later in the life cycle, other chemotherapy drugs damage the tumor cell's DNA, preventing it from reproducing.

Often, several chemotherapy drugs are used together in combination, so that cancer cells can be attacked simultaneously in a number of different ways.

Cytotoxic means "cell-killing," which describes how these anticancer drugs work—by killing cells. The cytotoxic drugs used in chemotherapy, though, are very selective in that they kill only rapidly growing cells, such as cancer cells.

However, many types of normal cells also grow rapidly, and unfortunately, these too are affected by these drugs, resulting in side effects. In fact, the drugs used in chemotherapy can be quite toxic to some people, leading to anemia and low white blood cell

counts, among other effects. With improvements in dosing schedules and in supportive care, many of the side effects have become
less of a problem.

Indications for Chemotherapy

Doctors use four guidelines to decide who is offered chemotherapy:

- Age under fifty years (premenopausal)
- Tumors that are hormone receptor–negative (more on this
  in Chapter 7)
- Tumor size larger than one inch (larger than two cm)
- Tumors with "aggressive" traits, such as high growth rate
  and poor histologic type

Women older than age fifty, or postmenopausal, usually have
similar results with hormonal therapy, which has fewer side effects
than chemotherapy. But the treatments are often combined with
others to gain the best advantage.

Controversies over Early-Stage, Node-Negative Cancers

For women with Stage I and II cancers whose cancer has *not*
spread to the lymph nodes, the need for chemotherapy is far less
certain. For a small group who have larger or fast-growing tumors,
the benefit seems clear. These women are believed to have a greater
chance of cancer recurrence, and adjuvant therapy can prevent
or delay its return.

However, women with the smallest tumors, less than half an
inch in size, are not as likely to have a recurrence after surgery and
radiation, and so they might opt not to have chemotherapy and
instead have hormone therapy, which has fewer side effects. Or

Neoadjuvant Chemotherapy

When it is given before the primary surgical treatment, chemotherapy is
termed "neoadjuvant" or "induction." For example, chemotherapy can
be given to shrink a tumor, which is then removed by surgery.

they may have neither. Each woman should discuss these treatment options with her doctor.

The Drugs

Primary Drugs

More than forty different drugs are active against breast cancer. Out of these, a handful are most effective and tend to be used more widely. These include:

Cyclophosphamide (Cytoxan)

Doxorubicin (Adriamycin)

Methotrexate

5-Fluorouracil (5-FU)

Vincristine (Oncovin)

Thiotepa

Doxorubicin (Adriamycin) is the single most effective agent in killing breast cancer cells, but it has many side effects. Cyclophosphamide also is widely effective, and it is less toxic than doxorubicin. These two drugs are the most commonly used of the chemotherapy agents.

Periwinkle Blue

Vincristine, one of the first-line chemotherapy drugs, is derived from the periwinkle plant, *Vinca rosea*. The drug is a member of a class of cytotoxic agents called plant alkaloids, all of which are derived from—as you might have guessed—the periwinkle plant. Despite their innocent appearance, these flowers provide some of the most powerful agents used to fight cancer.

Secondary Drugs

Chemotherapy does not work the same in everyone, and the first set of treatments may not control the cancer. For those women requiring a second round of treatment, another set of drugs may be used. These include:

Ifosfamide

Cisplatin

Etoposide

Mitomycin C

Vinblastine

Vinorelbine

Paclitaxel (Taxol)

Docetaxel (Taxotere)

These drugs are not as widely effective as the first group, but all of them have proven effective in many people with breast cancer, even when the primary drugs have failed.

Among these agents, Taxol, Taxotere, and vinorelbine are newer anticancer drugs. Taxol is made from the bark of the rare Pacific yew tree, and it takes several trees' worth of bark to yield enough drug for one person. But this drug can now be completely synthesized in the laboratory, so the short supply of yew trees is no longer a problem. Taxotere is a chemical cousin of Taxol that is extracted from the European yew tree. Both Taxol and Taxotere can have significant effects against recurrent or resistant breast cancer. Vinorelbine (Navelbine) is mainly used to treat lung cancer but also has shown some benefits in advanced breast cancer.

New Drugs

Many new drugs are in development and clinical testing. You or your doctor can consult the NCI's Cancer Information Service, which contains the latest results on each one. Their toll-free telephone number is 1-800-4-CANCER.

Supportive Therapy

Prednisone and leucovorin, though not cytotoxic drugs themselves, are given with many of the chemotherapy drugs to help reduce their side effects. Prednisone reduces inflammation and helps to prevent blood-related problems and gastrointestinal upset.

Leucovorin is given to provide the vitamin folic acid, which is necessary for normal cells but whose production is blocked by some chemotherapy drugs. In addition, this drug helps enhance the cancer-killing effect of 5-fluorouracil, with which it is often given.

Combination Chemotherapy

Although drugs such as cyclophosphamide and doxorubicin are very effective by themselves, extensive research has proven that combinations of these drugs are even more effective. Anywhere from *ten to one hundred times more* cancer cells are killed with combinations than with single-drug chemotherapy.

Generally two to four anticancer drugs are used together. The combinations are referred to by abbreviations, where the letters refer to the drugs included. The most widely used of these are:

CMF—cyclophosphamide (Cytoxan), methotrexate, and 5-fluorouracil

CAF (or FAC)—cyclophosphamide, doxorubicin (Adriamycin), and 5-fluorouracil

CA (or AC)—cyclophosphamide and doxorubicin (Adriamycin)

CMFP—cyclophosphamide, methotrexate, 5-fluorouracil, and prednisone

CMFVP—cyclophosphamide, methotrexate, 5-fluorouracil, vincristine, and prednisone

VATH—vinblastine, doxorubicin (Adriamycin), thiotepa, and fluoxymesterone

CMF is the most commonly used of the combinations, usually in women with early-stage disease. CAF is also widely used, particularly for women with larger tumors or more advanced cancers. CAF includes doxorubicin (the *A* stands for Adriamycin, the brand name of this drug), which is the strongest of the anticancer drugs but one with many side effects.

Many other combinations are under study—the variations seem endless—as experts continually mix and match the drugs looking for ways to improve the benefits and reduce the side effects.

Course of Therapy

Chemotherapy drugs are given for a few days, followed by several days to weeks when no treatment is given—this is called a *cycle*. Each drug is given on different days over the course of the cycle. Some drugs are given daily, some weekly, and some only once a month. These cycles then are repeated for anywhere from two to six months or up to one year in some cases. (In the past, chemotherapy had been given for up to four years!)

For example, in the CAF combination, cyclophosphamide is given every day for the first fourteen days of a four-week (twenty-eight-day) "cycle." Doxorubicin (Adriamycin) and 5-fluorouracil are given only on the first and eighth days of the month. During the second two weeks of the month, no treatment is given, while the person recovers her strength. Beginning on day 29, a new cycle starts. This same cycle is repeated every twenty-eight days for six cycles, lasting roughly six months.

In the regimen called FAC, the same three drugs are given, but on a different schedule. All three drugs are given on the first day, with 5-fluorouracil being repeated on the fourth or eighth day, followed by no therapy for two weeks. Beginning on day 21, a new cycle begins.

Adjuvant chemotherapy starts within two to six weeks after the initial surgery and does not overlap with the radiation treatments.

The question of whether chemotherapy should be given after surgery but *before* radiation therapy in breast-conserving therapy, especially in women at risk for metastatic disease, is being studied, but the results aren't clear yet. In advanced breast cancer, combination chemotherapy or hormonal therapy are often the first treatments given, followed by surgery and/or radiation and then more chemotherapy.

Why Does Chemotherapy Last So Long?

As fast as cancer cells divide, these cells also "rest" for periods between divisions, just like normal cells do. During these resting periods, the cancer cells are relatively safe from the chemotherapy drugs, which can only attack while the tumor cells are growing or dividing. Thus, chemotherapy is given over months to lessen the chance that "resting" cells left behind will "wake up" and cause a recurrence.

How Are the Drugs Administered?

Some chemotherapy drugs come in tablet form and are taken by mouth. These drugs can be taken at home.

Most anticancer drugs, though, must be given intravenously at the doctor's office, clinic, or outpatient center of the hospital. If many intravenous injections will be needed over a long time, the doctor may insert an *indwelling catheter*. A catheter is a tube that is surgically implanted into a major vein in the arm or chest. All injections are then given through this catheter.

The doses and schedules used for anticancer chemotherapy are carefully formulated to provide maximum benefit. To be effective, the drugs must be given at appropriate high doses and according to schedule. *It is the strength or intensity of the medicines that allows them to kill cancer cells.*

During treatment, your progress is checked regularly with blood tests, X rays, and physical examinations. If the side effects are too difficult to tolerate, the doses may be reduced. Medications also may be prescribed to reduce these side effects.

If the side effects cannot be adequately controlled, a new regimen may need to be substituted.

High-dose Chemotherapy and Bone Marrow Transplantation

Women with advanced cancer, those who have a high chance for cancer recurrence, and those whose cancers are unlikely to respond to regular chemotherapy may consider a new research treatment that combines very high doses of chemotherapy followed later by bone marrow transplantation. This treatment is experimental and only works for some women.

In this therapy, blood-forming cells are removed from the bone marrow or blood and are stored. These cells produce all the blood cells in the body, in-

Chemotherapy and the Older Woman

Contrary to what experts recommend, studies have shown that women over age sixty-five are less likely to be offered chemotherapy than younger women with the same stage of breast cancer. Furthermore, they may be given lower doses. But older women need and should receive full doses and full courses of chemotherapy, not reduced ones, to kill the cancer cells, just as in younger women.

cluding the white blood cells important in fighting infection and platelets that prevent bleeding. After removal of the bone marrow cells, the patient is given large doses of chemotherapy, which destroy the cancer and all of the remaining bone marrow as well. Later, the previously removed marrow cells are reinjected, and if all goes well, these regrow to restore the bone marrow to its normal strength, allowing the body to continue to produce blood cells and fight infection.

Caution: This is an experimental treatment that has severe effects of its own. Insurance company payment for this expensive, somewhat experimental procedure may also be a problem.

Side Effects and What to Do About Them

The anticancer drugs are all very potent, and each has its own set of side effects. Some women have relatively mild problems from their chemotherapy, but others have a more difficult course.

Although these side effects can be discouraging, it is important to remember that they occur because strong drugs are needed to destroy the cancer cells. Sometimes the doses or schedules can be changed somewhat to reduce the side effects, and sometimes medication can be prescribed to make these more tolerable.

Nausea and Vomiting

Most women who receive chemotherapy for breast cancer have some nausea and vomiting. This usually occurs within a few hours after taking the drugs and may last a day or two.

But these effects can be controlled or made milder in several ways:

- Antiemetic drugs can be given to prevent the nausea and vomiting. These include Zofran (ondansetron) and Kytril (granisetron), among others.
- Relaxation techniques can be taught to overcome some of the nausea.

- Eat smaller, more frequent meals and snacks, and avoid big meals and sweet, fried, or fatty foods.
- Avoid strong odors. Foods can be eaten cold or at room temperature to avoid their strong smells.

- Drink plenty of fluids, including cool, clear, unsweetened fruit juices such as apple juice and light sodas that are flat.
- Avoid alcohol.

The nausea is greatest right after treatment and may return each time the same drug is given. It may even occur in a few people before they receive a scheduled treatment with the drug, a condition called *anticipatory vomiting*.

Hair Loss

Hair loss occurs mostly with chemotherapy that includes the drug doxorubicin (Adriamycin). This hair loss may be complete, occurring on all parts of the body. Other drugs cause milder degrees of hair thinning. *But the hair will all grow back after treatment ends.* In the meantime, some strategies for coping with hair loss include the following:

- Be gentle to your hair. Use mild shampoos, soft hair brushes, no perms.
- Have your hair cut short, which will make it look fuller.
- Wear scarves or hats.
- Wear a wig.
- Use false eyelashes.

Anemia

Chemotherapy damages fast-growing cells, including the blood-forming cells of the bone marrow. The resulting *myelosuppression* can result in anemia, meaning there are too few red blood cells to deliver oxygen to all the body's tissues. The symptoms include tiredness, dizziness, and chills. To combat it:

- Get plenty of rest, and limit your activities.
- Eat a balanced diet, including iron-rich foods like spinach and red meat.
- *Ask* friends and family for help with home chores when you need it.
- Get up slowly from sitting or lying to avoid dizziness.

If anemia becomes a serious problem, your doctor may prescribe a drug called erythropoietin (Epogen), which helps correct anemia by stimulating the body to produce more red blood cells.

Infection

Chemotherapy reduces the body's ability to fight infection by damaging its white blood cells. These infections may occur anywhere in the body—the lungs, skin, urinary tract—and they don't heal as quickly. And simple infections can quickly become serious. To help prevent infection, you should:

- Avoid even minor scratches and scrapes, which may allow bacteria to enter the body. Use gloves when gardening; take care when using scissors, knives, or needles.
- Clean cuts promptly with soap and water, and use an antiseptic.
- Avoid people who have colds or other contagious infections, children who have been immunized recently, and crowds.
- Wash your hands often.

Antibiotics can cure most infections, especially if begun early. If you have a fever of 101°F for more than one hour, or for any other reason you suspect an infection is developing, report it to the doctor immediately.

Skin

The skin may become very dry during chemotherapy. Acne, rash, or blotchiness also may occur. Your doctor can recommend various lotions and creams to help with these problems. Cosmetics and makeups may also be tried to help cover any paleness or jaundice, should it develop.

The skin also may be overly sensitive to sunlight and easily sunburn. Protection from the sun with sunscreens, long-sleeved clothes, and hats is important.

Sometimes a rash or redness develops at the site of previous radiation therapy. This effect, called *radiation recall,* fades in hours or a day but should be reported to your doctor.

Some skin problems require immediate attention. If you feel burning or pain near the site of an IV injection, tell your doctor. Some drugs can damage tissues if they leak out during administration. Also, sudden or severe itching, hives, and rash, especially if wheezing or breathing difficulties occur, may be an allergic reaction and should be reported immediately.

Will You Be Able to Continue Working During Chemotherapy?
Most people receiving chemotherapy are able to continue working. Treatment sessions can be scheduled late in the day or before weekends so that they interfere as little as possible with work. All people suffer fatigue and need to limit activities or hours at work, so a part-time schedule may be better. More problematic are effects such as nausea or vomiting, which may prevent working for a day or so every cycle after receiving the drugs. Antiemetic drugs may be used to prevent or mollify this problem.

These side effects all vary from person to person, and even episode to episode. And they disappear entirely after treatment ends.

A *nurse oncologist* is available during all treatment sessions and can be an invaluable source of help and comfort in dealing with these side effects. A *support group* also can be a very good source of practical advice about coping with these problems. Talking with other women in the same circumstances reveals how others handle these problems.

Complications

With modern chemotherapy, long-term side effects are rare. Although most side effects cease after treatment ends, some late effects may persist.

- *Cardiotoxicity*—Heart damage may occur, particularly with the drugs doxorubicin (Adriamycin) and mitoxantrone (Novantrone).
- *Leukemia*—Rare.

• *Fertility problems*—Chemotherapy can damage the ovaries, and many women, especially those over age thirty-five, may not be able to become pregnant afterward.

It's Your Turn

1. Was cancer found in any of your lymph nodes?
   ❑   No
   ❑   Yes. How many? _____

2. Was the tumor positive or negative for estrogen receptors?
   ❑   Negative
   ❑   Positive*

*If you are over age fifty, you should discuss the possible use of hormone therapies with the doctor.

3. What chemotherapy regimen is planned or being used to treat your breast cancer?

_____

4. How long will it be given?
   ❑   2 months   ❑   4 months
   ❑   6 months   ❑   Other: _____

5. Are you using any medications to alleviate any nausea or vomiting?
   ❑   None needed
   ❑   Zofran
   ❑   Kytril
   ❑   Other: _____

6. Are you able to engage in most of your usual activities, without too much fatigue?
   ❑   Yes, mostly
   ❑   No
Which ones can't you do? _____

_____

7. What other side effects are you experiencing, and what are you doing about them?

_____

_____

_____

_____

8. Have you made any arrangements with family or friends to help out with daily chores?

❑   Yes

❑   No*

*You may have to *ask* friends or family for help if they don't offer.

9. Did you receive any immunizations or see your dentist be-fore starting chemotherapy?*

❑   Yes

❑   No

*Both infections and dental problems can be common during chemotherapy.

7

Hormonal Therapy

WHAT IS A HORMONE?

A hormone is a chemical produced naturally in the body by a gland, such as the adrenal gland. Hormones are secreted into the bloodstream and signal another part of the body to carry out a particular action. For example, the adrenal glands secrete adrenaline, which stimulates the heart to beat faster.

The hormone most important to breast cancer is *estrogen*. This hormone is produced by the ovaries each month during ovulation, as a regular part of the menstrual cycle. Among its other effects, estrogen prepares the breasts for pregnancy by stimulating growth of cells in the milk ducts and lobules.

But when breast cancer is present, estrogen also can stimulate the growth of the tumor cells. This is the basis for hormonal therapy.

What Is Hormonal Therapy?

Hormonal therapy (also called endocrine therapy) consists of giving a drug that acts on cells like a hormone. But in breast cancer, the drug's effect is opposite to estrogen's, actually blocking estrogen's path to the cancer cells.

In the treatment of breast cancer, the most widely used hormonal therapy is *tamoxifen*. Tamoxifen and similar drugs are synthetic, meaning they are made in the laboratory to interfere with the natural hormones.

Like chemotherapy, hormonal therapy is a systemic treatment, killing cancer cells throughout the body. Also like chemotherapy, it can be given as an *adjuvant* treatment, to kill cancer cells remaining after surgery and radiation and thereby prevent a recurrence of the cancer. Or it may be given as a *primary* therapy, by itself, without surgery, radiotherapy, or other drugs. Hormonal therapy alone may be used in advanced cancers, including recurrent or metastatic breast cancers.

Hormonal therapy is a much less intense treatment with far fewer side effects than chemotherapy, but it is just as effective as chemotherapy for many women, and even superior in some.

Who Gets Hormonal Therapy?

Just as with chemotherapy, there are several traits that doctors use to tell which women are likely to respond to hormonal therapy.

Estrogen Receptors

The main test for predicting if hormonal therapy will be effective is whether the tumor has estrogen receptors (hormone receptors) in its cells. Most breast tumors have estrogen receptors, which serve to attract estrogen and thereby help the tumor grow faster. All breast cancer cells start with estrogen receptors (termed *ER-positive*), but some tumors lose these during their development (become *ER-negative*).

Women with ER-positive cancers tend to respond well to hormonal therapy about 60 percent of the time, and those with ER-negative tumors respond better to chemotherapy. However, hormonal therapy still works in some ER-negative tumors.

The biopsy report tells if these receptors are present.

Progesterone Receptors
Progesterone is estrogen's hormone cousin in the ovulation cycle. The presence of receptors for progesterone in tumor cells (PR-positive) is a sign that the tumor may be responsive to hormonal therapy.

Menopausal Status

Of equal importance to estrogen receptors in the decision to use hormone therapy is a woman's age, or more specifically, whether she has passed the menopause.

In women over age fifty (postmenopausal), more tumors tend to be ER-positive and hormonal agents are more often effective. Even ER-negative cancers in these women may respond to these agents.

Women under age fifty (premenopausal) tend to respond better to chemotherapy and not as well to hormonal agents, since more of these women have ER-negative cancer.

Also in premenopausal women, the ovaries are still actively producing estrogen. Hormonal therapy may be needed to stop the ovaries and cut off this source of estrogen to the tumor.

Tumor Growth

Finally, the biopsy can determine if the tumor is fast-growing or slow-growing. Factors pointing to slow growth include small tumor size, certain tumor types, histologic grade I or II, and a low percentage of tumor cells in the "S-phase" of cell growth. Breast cancers having these features often respond to hormonal therapy.

So a complete biopsy report is important in deciding on hormonal therapy or chemotherapy. And now, a closer look at the particular uses of hormonal therapy.

Indications

Adjuvant Therapy in Early-stage Breast Cancer

Lymph Node–Positive Tumors: Women having evidence of cancer in their underarm lymph nodes receive adjuvant therapy, either chemotherapy or hormonal therapy, following their breast-conserving therapy (lumpectomy and radiation) or mastectomy. Hormonal therapy may be given to both postmenopausal and premenopausal women who have ER-positive tumors. And it works very well—as well as chemotherapy.

Some women having "high-risk" Stage II tumors, in whom the chance of spread is likely or suspected, may be offered hormonal therapy combined with chemotherapy.

Lymph Node–Negative Tumors: In the past, women without signs of cancer in their lymph nodes did not receive adjuvant treatment after the initial surgery and radiation. But, because of the chance of cancer recurrence, treatment is now usually offered.

Hormonal therapy, usually with tamoxifen, is the first choice for postmenopausal women with early-stage, ER-positive tumors. In premenopausal women, hormonal therapy is used only in those with cancers that are ER-positive.

Women having very small tumors, under half an inch in size, have a small chance of cancer recurring and may choose not to take any adjuvant treatment at all, but tamoxifen is being used more in an adjuvant role in these women.

Tamoxifen also is being evaluated in research studies for its effectiveness in women with ductal carcinoma in situ, the earliest stage of breast cancer.

Advanced-stage Breast Cancer

For women with advanced disease, including metastatic and recurrent cancer, hormonal therapy may be given alone as primary therapy or combined with chemotherapy and other forms of treatment. Sometimes, the chemotherapy is given first (neoadjuvant or induction treatment), before surgery or radiation, with hormonal therapy being given afterward. Again, women whose tumors are ER-positive are more likely to respond to hormonal therapy.

Among premenopausal women with ER-positive tumors, hormonal therapy can be given to stop the ovaries from producing estrogen. This can be achieved with drugs, such as tamoxifen or the LHRH analogues, as well as with surgery.

Metastatic Cancer: When breast cancer has spread to other areas of the body (metastatic cancer), hormonal therapy may be given as the first treatment. Or it may be combined with chemotherapy.

Chemotherapy, with or without hormonal therapy, is offered to most patients with ER-negative tumors or with disease involving organs such as the liver, lungs, or brain.

Recurrent Cancer: Women who develop a recurrence of cancer after treatment for the first one may consider hormonal therapy to slow or stop the cancer's spread, especially those with ER-positive tumors. Tamoxifen is the first-choice treatment for these women, the other hormonal therapies being used if the tumor does not respond to tamoxifen or when it has begun to progress despite tamoxifen. Women who have previously responded to hormonal therapy or have had several years since their primary cancer tend to respond better to hormonal therapy.

Easier But Just As Effective

Because hormonal therapy is an "easier" treatment than chemotherapy—that is, it has few side effects and is often easier to administer—it should not be considered any less effective or any "less" of a treatment. Studies have compared hormonal therapy directly against chemotherapy, and in the groups of women for whom hormonal therapy is indicated, it has equal or better results compared to chemotherapy.

The Drugs

The first hormonal treatment that was used in breast cancer was not a drug—it was surgery to remove the ovaries (oophorectomy). By taking out the gland that produces estrogen, it effectively stopped estrogen's flow to the cancer, and the tumor shrank in many cases. This became the basis for using hormonal drugs to fight breast cancer.

Today, tamoxifen is the major hormonal agent used in this fight. The other agents tend to cause more side effects than tamoxifen, but when a woman's breast cancer doesn't respond to tamoxifen or if her disease progresses while on tamoxifen, the other agents can still work. In fact, hormonal therapies are used sequentially, with a new one introduced when resistance to the initial drug develops.

And all still cause fewer side effects than chemotherapy.

Tamoxifen

Tamoxifen citrate (Nolvadex) is called an *antiestrogen drug,* which describes how it works. It blocks the tumor from using estrogen by filling up the estrogen receptors in the tumor. Fewer "parking places" for the real estrogen means less gets to the tumor, slowing or stopping the tumor's growth and, in some cases, causing death of the cancer cells. Because tamoxifen also can work in ER-negative tumors, it probably interferes with cancer cells' growth in other ways, too.

Indications: Tamoxifen has been used since the 1970s to treat *advanced breast cancer* in postmenopausal women and, since 1989, premenopausal women as well. It can induce a remission or shrinkage of the tumor in more than half of these women. And it can produce a response regardless of a woman's lymph node status or her tumor's ER status. The greatest advantage, however, tends to be seen in women who have evidence of cancer in their lymph nodes and who have ER-positive tumors.

Tamoxifen also is used as an adjuvant therapy, after surgery and/or radiation, to prevent recurrence of cancer in *early-stage breast cancer*. It is used routinely in postmenopausal women but again is effective in selected premenopausal women as well. Study results show that tamoxifen reduces the risk of cancer recurring by 25 percent in these women. It also reduces, by 39 percent, the chances of a new breast cancer.

Finally, tamoxifen can delay the recurrence of breast cancer and prolong the lives of women with breast cancer.

Tamoxifen and Its Secondary Effects

Postmenopausal women typically have progressive bone loss (osteoporosis) and a higher risk of heart disease that increases with age, because of the loss of "protective" estrogen with the menopause. Despite tamoxifen's anti-estrogen effects on breast cancer cells, it does not cause further harm in these two areas.

Course of Therapy: Tamoxifen comes in tablet form and is taken at home, every day, just like any other prescription drug. Typically 20 mg, one or two tablets, is taken orally (by mouth) every day. The treatment can last for five years or more.

Treatment begins soon after surgery or radiation, usually within two to six weeks in early-stage breast cancer, but this varies for advanced disease.

Following the start of tamoxifen in metastatic cancer, an unusual "flare" reaction may occur. This consists of an apparent worsening of symptoms, such as bone pain and an increase in tumor size. In addition, it may produce an excess of calcium in the blood (hypercalcemia), resulting in nausea, fatigue, muscle weakness, and confusion—symptoms that should be reported to the doctor. This reaction fades after a few days to weeks and is considered by some to be a good sign that tamoxifen is working.

The "flare" reaction can be seen after starting some other hormonal therapies also, such as estrogens and androgen. Tamoxifen and other hormonal treatments are generally continued for as long as the disease remains under control in those with metastatic disease.

Side Effects: Tamoxifen causes few side effects, and these are generally mild. The most frequent problems are *menopausal symptoms*—hot flashes, vaginal dryness and irritation, and irregular periods—seen in premenopausal women. There may be some abnormal vaginal bleeding or discharge, which should be reported to the doctor. Another drug may be given to help reduce the hot flashes if necessary, and a lubricant may be needed during sexual activity.

Other rare side effects include blurred vision, nausea or stomach upset, skin rash, mood changes, weight gain, and blood clots. If any of these effects is noticed, it can be discussed with the doctor.

Fewer than 5 percent of women have to stop taking tamoxifen because of intolerable or severe side effects.

Sex, the Younger Woman, and Tamoxifen

Despite tamoxifen's menopausal-like side effects, it does not decrease a woman's fertility. So premenopausal women *must* be careful about getting pregnant—but don't take birth control pills! Your doctor can advise about which methods of contraception to use during tamoxifen therapy.

Uterine Cancer: Tamoxifen can stimulate growth of the cells lining the uterus, and with this growth comes a small risk of cancer. Doctors can check for this through regular gynecologic exams. Women should report any unusual spotting or vaginal discharge, menstrual irregularities, or pelvic pain or pressure to their doctor.

Fear of uterine cancer should *not* be a reason to avoid tamoxifen if a woman has breast cancer. Uterine cancer is more easily treated than breast cancer, and despite the increased risk, very few women will develop this problem because of tamoxifen—about one in 1,000 women with breast cancer develop uterine cancer yearly versus about two to three per 1,000 who take tamoxifen. In contrast, the benefits of tamoxifen against breast cancer are clear and significant, and these more than offset the risks.

Tamoxifen Information

The manufacturer of Nolvadex has set up the Zeneca Breast Cancer Patient Education Service, which provides a complimentary educational video and information on breast cancer and tamoxifen: 1-800-34-LIFE4 (1-800-345-4334)

Other Antiestrogen Drugs

Tamoxifen, though by far the most widely used, is not the only drug in this class. Toremifene, droloxifene, idoxifene, and others also work by blocking estrogen's access to cancer cells. Their roles and effectiveness are still being determined in clinical studies.

Progestins

Megestrol acetate (Megace) and medroxyprogesterone acetate (Provera), the two main progestins, are second-line agents, used when tamoxifen is no longer effective. They are useful in women having advanced breast cancer, especially postmenopausal women. The response rate is comparable to tamoxifen's, but there are more side effects.

One frequent side effect is weight gain, which can be significant. Up to 35 percent of women treated with these drugs gain more than twenty pounds, due primarily to an increased appetite brought on by these drugs.

Megestrol acetate requires 160 mg a day, given orally as one tablet four times each day. Medroxyprogesterone acetate can be taken once daily, but it requires a dose of at least 500 mg a day, meaning many pills (ten or more) must be swallowed.

Aminoglutethimide and Aromatase Inhibitors

Aromatase is an enzyme that helps produce estrogen in fat tissues, muscle, and the liver. It can also be found in breast tumors.

These nonovarian sites can be sources of estrogen for breast cancer cells in postmenopausal women.

The aromatase inhibitor drugs block this enzyme to prevent production of estrogen. They are useful as a second-line therapy in postmenopausal women with advanced breast cancer whose disease has progressed despite tamoxifen. Premenopausal women whose ovaries have been removed or stopped by radiation (ablation) or chemotherapy may also be candidates.

Aminoglutethimide: Aminoglutethimide (Cytadren) suppresses the adrenal gland, which produces the chemicals that are ultimately converted by aromatase into estrogen. Unfortunately, these chemicals are also necessary for other purposes, and an additional drug must be taken to replace them in patients taking aminoglutethimide.

In clinical studies, aminoglutethimide produces responses in up to 35 percent of women with advanced cancer. A response is more likely in those with ER-positive tumors.

The drug is administered in a dose of 1000 mg a day, given as one 250-mg tablet four times each day. Hydrocortisone also must be taken with it to replace other blocked hormones.

Anastrozole: Anastrozole (Arimidex) is a new "selective" aromatase inhibitor, which blocks production of estrogen only. Thus, it has fewer side effects than the other drugs in this class.

It is indicated for treatment of postmenopausal women with advanced breast cancer whose disease has progressed despite tamoxifen. But because it is generally well tolerated, it may be considered as an alternative to megestrol acetate and other hormonal agents for second-line treatment.

In clinical trials, anastrozole showed clinical benefits in 35 percent of patients, a rate comparable to that achieved with megestrol acetate. Patients who did not respond to tamoxifen previously or who had ER-negative tumors were unlikely to respond to anastrozole.

An important advantage of anastrozole is its excellent tolerability. In particular, weight gain, which is a common problem with megestrol acetate, occurs in far fewer patients. Other side effects of anastrozole are uncommon and include fatigue or weakness (16 percent), nausea or diarrhea (15.6 percent), headache (13 percent), hot flashes (12 percent), and pain (10.7 percent).

Anastrozole comes in 1-mg tablets, which are taken orally once each day.

LHRH Analogues

Luteinizing hormone-releasing hormone (LHRH, or gonadotropin-releasing hormone, GnRH) is produced naturally by the body to help control the ovulation cycle. Synthetic versions of the natural hormone have been produced—goserelin (Zoladex), leuprolide (Lupron), buserelin, and triptorelin—which block ovarian function and stop its production of estrogen. Menses generally cease within two or three months after starting this therapy but will restart on its withdrawal.

In clinical studies, goserelin (the only one of the LHRH analogues approved for use in breast cancer) achieved a response similar to that obtained with surgical removal of the ovaries—about 36 percent of patients had slowing or control of tumor growth or improvement in its symptoms. Thus, it provides an alternative to surgical removal of the ovaries or to tamoxifen-induced suppression of the ovaries.

The LHRH analogues are indicated in the treatment of advanced breast cancer in pre- or perimenopausal women in whom the ovaries are still functioning to produce estrogen.

Side effects are mild and generally well tolerated. The most common ones include hot flashes and other menopausal symptoms.

Goserelin is given as an injection once monthly in the doctor's office. The tumor "flare" reaction, as described with tamoxifen, is seen in about a quarter of users on starting therapy. Although menstrual periods stop during treatment, birth control is necessary for the duration of treatment and for twelve weeks afterward.

Androgens

Though not commonly used, the androgen fluoxymesterone (Halotestin) can be given as a third-line treatment for postmenopausal women with ER-positive advanced or recurrent breast cancer. It is effective in about 20 percent of patients and sometimes is combined with chemotherapy.

Androgens are "male" hormones and result in masculiniza-tion—loss or thinning of scalp hair, increased facial and body hair, acne, deepening voice, and other virilizing traits. Menstrual irregu-larities and changes in libido are also seen.

Estrogens

Diethylstilbestrol (DES) and others estrogens operate very dif-ferently from the antiestrogen therapies. They *increase* the body's level of estrogen, and, opposite to what you would think, these very high levels can cause tumors to shrink. But the estrogens are used very rarely because of their high frequency of side effects.

Antiprogestins

Mifepristone—or RU-486, the French abortion pill—has been in the news for reasons not related to breast cancer. But it inhibits breast cancer cells' growth by blocking estrogen's cousin, proges-terone. However, the drug has more side effects than other hor-monal drugs. It was approved in 1993 for use in treatment of ad-vanced breast cancers.

Ovarian Surgery

Finally, back to the "original" hormone therapy, which still has a role today, though a small one. Premenopausal women who have advanced cancers that are ER-positive may consider surgical re-moval of their ovaries (oophorectomy). This treatment causes the tumors to shrink in about one-third of cases. However, the same results can be achieved with LHRH analogues, without the com-plications of surgery.

Surgery to remove other estrogen-producing glands, such as the adrenal, is rarely done today. If necessary, drugs can be given to medically stop these glands.

It's Your Turn

1. Did your biopsy report indicate that your tumor was positive or negative for hormone receptors? Which ones?
   - ❑ Estrogen receptor–positive
   - ❑ Estrogen receptor–negative
   - ❑ Progesterone receptor–positive
   - ❑ Progesterone receptor–negative

2. Which hormonal agent have you been prescribed?
   _____
   Why this one? _____
   _____

3. How long will you take tamoxifen?
   ❑ 5 years   ❑ more than 5 years

4. If you are premenopausal, are you using birth control while taking tamoxifen or LHRH analogues? Which kind?*
   - ❑ Condoms, diaphragm*
   - ❑ Birth control pills
   - ❑ None

*The only correct answer. Birth control pills contain estrogen and should not be taken by a woman who has had breast cancer.

5. Have you noticed any side effects from your hormonal therapy?
   - ❑ Menopausal symptoms—hot flashes, vaginal irritation and dryness, irregular periods
   - ❑ Weight gain (especially with megestrol acetate)
   - ❑ Swelling of the limbs, or fluid retention
   - ❑ Nausea, vomiting
   - ❑ Drowsiness, lethargy
   - ❑ Depression, mood changes
   - ❑ Calf pain or shortness of breath*

*Blood clots are a serious problem that may occur rarely with several of the hormonal drugs. These symptoms should be reported immediately to the doctor.

6. Have you had any unusual vaginal bleeding while taking tamoxifen?

☐ No

☐ Yes*

*You should report this to your doctor, because tamoxifen may cause a slightly increased risk for uterine cancer.

8

How Are You Doing?

During Treatment: Ups and Downs

IN THE MONTHS after surgery, your treatment will continue with chemotherapy, radiotherapy, and/or hormonal therapy according to your personal needs. The long treatments are needed to beat the cancer, but often at a high physical cost to your body.

Also occurring during this period are anxiety, anger, and depression. These are the emotional reactions to the changes in your life caused by the cancer and its treatment.

During treatment, these physical and emotional "side effects" may interfere, preventing you from doing many of the things you want to do or usually do. Some days are much worse than others. You won't be prevented from doing everything, but it will not be possible for you to keep up with all of your regular routine.

Over the next few months, you will have to find ways to balance your usual activities with what the treatment allows you. By planning your time more carefully and relying on family and friends for help and support, you should find it is possible to cope well with the challenges of this period.

Dealing with the Physical Effects

For the first time in the course of this disease, you may actually feel ill, due to the side effects of radiation or adjuvant therapy.

Fatigue, one of the most common side effects, is seen with both radiotherapy and chemotherapy and results from the treatment's effects on the healthy cells of the body. Hot flashes, skin changes, and symptoms of menopause can be caused by hormonal treatments. These as well as nausea, vomiting, loss of appetite, hair loss, and infections can occur with chemotherapy.

The side effects are uncomfortable, but tolerable. Some, like nausea, can be controlled with medication. But the effects last as long as you receive treatments.

The result is, you feel run down and weaker—and vulnerable. This can be disturbing for a person who is used to being healthy.

What Can Be Done?

During treatments, you should talk to the doctor or nurse about any side effects you are having, as well as ones to watch for. They can suggest ways to avoid or lessen these problems and maybe prescribe some medication or even changes to your treatment plan, if necessary.

There are also some things you can do yourself to control these problems. Simple changes in your diet, a little exercise, and even relaxation exercises can help.

What Does a Change in Treatments Mean?

In a few people, side effects become intolerable enough for your doctor to change the treatment plan. Several options are possible, including these:

- Delay a scheduled treatment to allow your body time to recover
- Reduce the dose of drug
- Switch the treatment to a new combination of drugs

All of these options are safe, and they do not necessarily reduce the effectiveness of the treatments you are receiving or mean that treatments aren't working. Many drugs are effective against breast cancer, but they affect people differently. Sometimes it is simply a matter of selecting treatments that don't have so many side effects for you.

Is the Treatment Working?

During the treatments, you will be monitored with a series of blood tests and X rays. These tests are the only way to learn whether a treatment is producing the desired effect. Not all treatments work the same for everyone. Switching to another treatment using different drugs might kill more cancer cells.

Dealing with the Emotional Effects

Any serious health problem can bring major changes to a person's life, threatening your sense of well-being, disrupting daily schedules, and straining personal relationships. In the weeks after surgery, many women will have periods of anxiety, anger, crying, and other unsettling emotions. These feelings are natural responses to having cancer and to the changes caused by the treatments.

And there are ways that you can plan to cope if they do occur.

Changes in Body Image

A mastectomy or any breast surgery is traumatic. In our society, breasts are symbols of femininity and sexuality, and women who lose a breast understandably may worry about their appearance or "completeness" as a woman. Likewise, the hair loss that accompanies some chemotherapy, although temporary, can be upsetting because it affects a person's outward appearance.

Despite the fears, neither a mastectomy nor hair loss will prevent a woman from resuming the same close relationship with her partner, including sex, as before. Talking with your partner about your concerns—and also to other women who have had breast cancer—can be reassuring.

Anxiety and Depression

Aside from affecting your sense of body image, cancer also evokes a wide range of strong emotions, from anger to fear to depression. Concerns about family, feelings of loneliness, and just uncertainty about the future are common.

These feelings in turn may lead to insomnia, loss of appetite, and less exercise, making you feel physically tired, weak, and more out of sorts. The side effects from radiation and chemotherapy can also contribute to these problems.

> **Look Good . . . Feel Better**
> This program, run by the American Cancer Society, helps women receiving cancer treatment learn about using makeups, cosmetics, hairstyles, and other beauty techniques to make themselves feel better about their appearance during this time. Call 1-800-395-LOOK or your local ACS chapter for information.

These emotions are understandable and normal. But they can be made better if you employ some simple coping strategies:

- Talk about your feelings with loved ones.
- Visit your friends.
- Get some exercise—nothing beats a nice walk outdoors.
- Allow people to do things for you, such as make meals or do errands.
- Reward yourself with at least one pleasure a day, such as a meal or movie.
- Do something different that you've always wanted to do.

Reminding yourself of the goals of treatment can help you keep a positive outlook on days when the going gets tough. Also, sharing fears and feelings with family or friends makes many people feel better. Talking allows others to show their concern and offer their support.

Visiting support groups and talking with other women who have had breast cancer will let you share ideas with other women in your situation. Your nurses and doctors also will answer questions as well as give reassurance. And counselors or therapists may be consulted.

Some simple changes in daily activities—the same ones that help limit the physical side effects of therapy—can work to reduce the emotional effects, too.

Would Prozac Help?
Periods of anxiety and depression are perfectly normal responses to having breast cancer. If the problems are intense or if they continue after treatment ends, a short session with a psychologist or psychiatrist can go a long way. A brief treatment with an antidepressant medication also may help.

Taking Care of Yourself

Rather than wait for the physical side effects or depression to happen, you can do things in your daily routine that will prevent or lessen some of these effects.

Diet

A balanced diet with adequate protein and calories can help fend off weakness and fatigue, repair damaged tissues, and help protect the immune system. And it improves a person's sense of well-being. In fact, you need to eat *more* calories than before to help your body rebuild and heal.

Some guidelines to help you maintain good nutrition during cancer treatment are:

- Eat according to a schedule, rather than as you feel like it.

- To avoid overfilling, eat smaller, more frequent meals and snacks.

- Eat a balanced diet, including the daily minimums of protein, fruits and vegetables, and bread or grain products.

- To increase your energy, *add extra calories.* Try mayonnaise, butter, cream, cream cheese, sauces, and all those other forbidden treats on foods.

- *Add extra protein* by snacking on diet supplement drinks (milkshakes) or crackers with cheese or peanut butter.

A short walk half an hour before dinner can stimulate a poor appetite; avoiding liquids before meals prevents early filling; and keeping a selection of foods on hand adds variety. On those days after chemotherapy when cooking may be a problem, rely on friends or family for help. Or prepare some meals beforehand.

A simple, balanced diet is all you need. Macrobiotics and other cancer-fighting fad diets are a waste of money.

Exercise

Though you may feel you need it just because of that high-cal diet, exercise is in itself an important part of the treatment plan.
Staying physically fit helps maintain strength and stamina, combats depression, and bolsters self-esteem. It helps your appetite, helps you to relax, and helps you sleep. Also, it gets you out and doing something, away from the anxiety. All of these help you to recover faster.

This exercise is nothing terribly complicated. Two kinds are called for in the "exercise prescription":

Arm Exercises: After surgery, simple arm exercises, called *range-of-motion exercises*, will keep your arm from becoming stiff, which can happen when scar tissue forms in the muscles following a mastectomy or surgery. A physical therapist will show you these exercises, which are just a series of ordinary arm movements. The exercises are done for ten minutes at a time, three times a day.

Exercising starts slowly and gently and may even be done in bed right after surgery:

- Clenching the hand into a fist and relaxing, or squeezing a rubber ball

- Brushing and combing your hair

- Moving the arm through its normal arc, or range of motion

Gradually, exercising becomes more active and can include such things as:

- Raising and stretching the arms overhead, or back scratching

- Wall walking or climbing with your fingers

- Rope turning (as in jump rope)

A second goal of arm exercises is to prevent *lymphedema*, which is the swelling in the arm that can occur after lymph nodes are removed from the underarm. If lymphedema occurs, these same exercises, done more intensively, can help relieve it.

Managing Lymphedema

Arm swelling can develop suddenly following surgery and can be difficult to control. Range-of-motion arm exercises, done intensively, can help relieve lymphedema if it occurs. Other strategies to reduce it include support sleeves or elastic compression sleeves, "lymph drainage" massage, and pneumatic pumps. Some physical therapists even specialize in this problem. The National Lymphedema Network (1-800-541-3259) offers support and more information.

Weight-bearing Exercise: For the next set of exercises, you will have to get out of bed. Because of the fatigue from radiation and chemotherapy, your body naturally wants to rest, but this inactivity can cause your muscles to waste. This causes you to have even less energy and strength.

The weight in weight-bearing exercise is not barbells—just your own weight—and it simply means moving about *actively*. It can include exercising to an aerobics video on TV, or using stationary bikes or stair climbers, or enrolling in a class at the health club. Tennis and running also count, but to start, simple *brisk* walking can be done for at least half an hour every other day.

> **Exercise at the Y**
> The YWCA sponsors an exercise and peer-support program called ENCORE-PLUS that is specifically designed for women with breast cancer. Contact your local branch for information.

Relaxation and Stress Management

Just as a good diet and exercise can limit side effects of treatment and speed your recovery, some other simple "exercises" can ensure your emotional health during this period:

- Muscle tension and release
- Rhythmic breathing
- Visualization or imagery
- Distraction
- Biofeedback

The doctor or nurse can explain these techniques to you. Many other ways are used to control anxiety—personal faith and devotion, meditation, massage, hypnosis, support groups, or even stress-management tapes. No one way works for everyone, and the point is simply to find one that works well for you.

Coping with Other People's Reactions

Despite all that's been said, there are still limits to your energies during this time, and you will need to rely on the people around you for extra help and support.

Your illness is changing the lives of others, too. Over the months of treatment, their fears and feelings are bound to appear, and these need to be understood.

Family

During times of crisis, families come together. But changes can be hard to handle for them too, and even the strongest families have their bad moments.

Children may express their fears by misbehaving. Trying to keep illness hidden from younger children may only increase their fears about what they suspect is some terrible secret. They should be told whatever they are old enough to understand, along with assurances that Mommy will get better and is still there for them.

Some teenagers are able physically to do extra housework but psychologically may be too young for the added responsibility. They may resent doing the mother's work at an age when they are trying to identify themselves apart from the family. Drinking, drugs, and other misbehaviors may occur. Again, being open and talking about the problems are helpful. Be careful not to expect too much from teenagers.

Husbands or partners may suffer stress from the uncertainty, financial pressures, and feelings of neglect or guilt. And then there is the question of sex. There are a multitude of opportunities for misinterpretations and hurt feelings between partners. Open communication and planning with the partner—and sometimes a little massage—help. Divorces happen, but uncommonly, and probably in marriages that were weak in the first place.

If problems become severe, short-term family counseling may be a good idea.

Friends

True friends should be relied on to lend comfort and courage. Sometimes, though, *you* may have to make the first move. Friends may feel awkward about not knowing what to say, how to say it, or what to do. You can help relieve their fears by talking openly and assuring them that no matter what they say, their caring is what counts.

Fellow Workers

At work, some women enjoy the support from a few close friends, whereas others choose not to tell any of their coworkers about their illness. Insurance forms can be filed confidentially through the personnel office, and the only person who may need to know is your supervisor, if extra time off is needed.

As with family, if misunderstandings arise, open communication should assure coworkers and employers that you will be back at full speed very soon. Keeping up contacts with others at work during your treatment is a good way to avoid later problems.

Can You Work During Treatments?
Many women do. You may need to take some time off, as little as a few hours for treatment sessions or some whole days when the side effects are at their worst. If fatigue becomes too great, you can ask to work part time for a period. The federal Family and Medical Leave Act of 1993 insures time off for workers with a major illness, providing up to twelve weeks per year of unpaid leave, with benefits intact.

Social Life

Among casual friends and social groups, many women fear that they will be rejected or left out because of their disease. Loss of self-esteem is common following breast surgery, which can lead to self-consciousness in groups. Among all groups of people, there will be some who are fearful or misinformed, and others who simply do not know what to say. Being open and dealing positively with your illness will help others understand how *they* should feel and act as well.

If your friends are not available as often as you would like, try getting out by yourself, if only for a short walk or a shopping trip. Recreation helps to relieve tension, and being out in a change of scenery and among people, will help lift your spirits.

Keeping busy means that there is less time to sit idle and worry about uncertainties and fears.

Support Groups

Friends and family, no matter how caring, sometimes cannot replace the empathy you feel when talking with another woman who has had breast cancer. Support groups can help by letting you see how others cope with their jobs, changing family roles, household duties, children's fears, insurance problems, and friends who don't know what to do or say. Women who participate in these groups often become less anxious, less depressed, and less afraid.

However, different women seek different help from these groups, and some may prefer individual counseling. You may try several groups before finding one that fits. The hospital likely has its own breast cancer support group, but the American Cancer Society also keeps a listing of these for every area. There are support groups for spouses and family, too.

Reach to Recovery

Reach to Recovery is a program of the American Cancer Society that is staffed by volunteers who have had mastectomies or breast cancer themselves. These volunteers visit women before and during treatment to discuss physical, emotional, and even cosmetic concerns. Having overcome the many challenges posed by breast cancer, they offer positive role models and invaluable practical experience. Your local ACS chapter has information on this program.

    ## It's Your Turn

1. Are you having any physical side effects from treatments?
   - ❏ Fatigue
   - ❏ Skin rash (with radiation)
   - ❏ Nausea or vomiting (with chemotherapy)
   - ❏ Loss of appetite (with chemotherapy)
   - ❏ Increased appetite (with tamoxifen)
   - ❏ Hair loss (with chemotherapy)
   - ❏ Hot flashes, skin changes (with tamoxifen, some chemotherapy)

2. How are you doing emotionally? Rate your feelings from 1 to 5 (with 5 being often or always, 3 being sometimes, and 1 being rarely or never).*

<table>
<tr><td>Depressed, listless:</td><td>(often) 5 4 3 2 1 (rarely)</td></tr>
<tr><td>Anxious, fearful, restless:</td><td>5 4 3 2 1</td></tr>
<tr><td>Angry:</td><td>5 4 3 2 1</td></tr>
<tr><td>Fearful of going out, seeing friends:</td><td>5 4 3 2 1</td></tr>
<tr><td>Crying spells:</td><td>5 4 3 2 1</td></tr>
<tr><td>Frequently changing moods:</td><td>5 4 3 2 1</td></tr>
</table>

*Talking a few times with a counselor, psychologist, or psychiatrist may help calm these disturbing feelings.

3. Are you able to talk about your illness and feelings with family and friends? With whom?

❑ Husband
❑ Sister or other family
❑ Adult daughter
❑ Best friend
❑ Support group

4. Do you have a regular exercise program?

❑ Aerobics video or TV show
❑ Stair climber or stationary bike
❑ Running
❑ Aerobics class at a health center or gym
❑ Dance class
❑ Walking
❑ Other: _____

How often do you do this exercise? _____

5. Are family and friends helping out with household chores and errands?

❑ Yes
❑ No*

*Sometimes you may have to ask them directly to help with a specific errand.

9

After Treatment

THE CHEMOTHERAPY has ended. So has the nausea.

Your appetite has returned. If your hair has fallen out, it is now filling in. And within the next few weeks, you'll have enough energy for tennis, dancing, or whatever makes you happy.

The rigors of the last few months of therapy for breast cancer will soon be behind you. But there are some lingering effects that may need attention.

Foremost, it is vitally important that you continue to take special care of yourself and see your doctor regularly. There also may be some recurring feelings of anxiety or depression. And there are the people around you—family, friends, and coworkers—who, though well-meaning, may have some confusing feelings toward you as a result of your illness. These will need some attention as well.

Follow-up Care

After the treatments end, each of the doctors who treated you— the surgeon, radiation oncologist, medical oncologist, and the plastic surgeon if you had breast reconstruction—will want to see you at least once more. One of these doctors, whichever one you prefer, will see you regularly for awhile.

For the next two years, there are appointments for physical exams and blood tests every two to four months. Mammograms and maybe some extra scans will be done every six to twelve months, as the doctor closely follows your recovery and watches carefully for signs of cancer recurrence. After the second year, if all is going well, the checkups become much less frequent, perhaps only once a year.

If you are taking tamoxifen, your gynecologist will want to see you at least yearly for a pelvic exam and Pap smear. If you have any unusual vaginal bleeding or discharge, or other symptoms, you will need to be seen sooner.

At home, you should examine both breasts monthly for lumps or rashes. Also check for lumps in the arm or neck. Persistent symptoms of any kind—cough, shortness of breath, abdominal or bone pain—should be reported.

Because you have had cancer before, your chances of getting it again are slightly higher, and it is something you should help your doctor watch for.

Initially, all the everyday aches and pains may seem alarming, but gradually they'll become less noticeable. Certainly don't hesitate to have them checked if you are concerned or if they persist.

If the Cancer Returns

For some women, the cancer does not totally disappear after the first bout of treatments. Hidden disease can reappear up to thirty years later, but most often it happens in the first two or three years. It may recur in the same breast, the opposite healthy breast, or elsewhere in the body.

Treatment options for a recurrence are the same as for the original tumor. Recurrent cancers can be treated and controlled, though they usually do not disappear. Women sometimes live with these for twenty and more years. Much of the research being done on breast cancer is focused on finding new and better treatments for such recurrences.

Gearing back up for another fight can be very tough emotionally. But women who have been through it once have the advantage of knowing what to expect, and they also have already developed their coping strategies.

Getting Things Back to Normal

The two periods of greatest emotional stress for people with cancer are just after the diagnosis, as you would expect, but also immediately after treatment ends. Leaving the routine in which doctors, nurses, even friends and family are constantly watching over and caring for you isn't necessarily easy, which you wouldn't expect. There is relief at having finished the treatments, but there may also be anxiety as you get back in step with the usual routine and people.

Your Feelings

Feelings of anxiety, fear, anger, and depression are common at this time. Emotional upset is experienced by most people after cancer, but it usually decreases with time. The coping strategies used during the treatments, as outlined in Chapter 8, can be relied on again here. These include:

- Talking openly about fears or expectations with your family or friends
- Using relaxation techniques to reduce stress
- Seeing friends and planning to do enjoyable activities
- Attending support groups for cancer survivors

Sharing your thoughts and feelings with loved ones can help everyone feel more at ease. It also opens the way for others to show their concern and offer support again. The worries fade eventually as you rejoin your old routine and activities.

Your doctor or nurse again can suggest ways to speed up this process of emotional healing.

Sexuality

When a woman learns she has breast cancer, one of her initial concerns is how this will affect her sexual activity. Fatigue and illness from chemotherapy and radiation treatments can limit desire for sexual contact during treatment, as well as make it uncomfortable. But after treatment ends, you will probably want to resume your sex life.

Having a mastectomy or lumpectomy should not affect your sense of pleasure or your partner's. Getting started may be more of a problem as a change in body often causes self-consciousness and fear of rejection. The partner may feel hesitant for various reasons, including a fear of hurting you.

Talking openly with your partner will be the first step in reconfirming what you already knew anyway: that your breast was not the only attractive thing about you. And it will avoid misunderstanding and fear on both sides. Sometimes, simple hugging or

Dyspareunia Is What Doctors Call It

If hormonal treatments continue to cause vaginal dryness, this can make sexual intercourse painful (dyspareunia). Using a lubricant may help, or your doctor can prescribe a cream product to use.

other "baby steps" may be a good start toward both of you feeling ready again.

Breast Reconstruction

Reconstruction of the breast helps many women regain a positive sense of body image and attractiveness, and with it self-esteem and confidence. If this was not performed during the initial surgery, reconstruction using tissue flaps or implants can be performed at a later point when you and your doctor agree.

Coping with Menopausal Symptoms

Chemotherapy may induce an early menopause. The symptoms are the same as those of natural menopause—hot flashes, headaches, vaginal dryness, irritability. And they can actually be more intense than usually experienced in natural menopause.

Understanding that these effects may occur can help in preparing for them. Stress management or relaxation techniques also may help, or your doctor may prescribe vitamins or medication to lessen the discomfort.

Estrogen-replacement therapy, which is often prescribed for postmenopausal women to ease the discomforts of menopause, is not used after breast cancer because the active ingredient, estrogen, can act as a stimulant for growth of any remaining cancer cells. Even so-called "traditional" or herbal remedies may contain estrogen and therefore should not be used without the doctor's approval.

Tamoxifen, though it usually does *not* cause menopause, can cause menopause-like symptoms. Women taking this drug should be careful to use birth control methods (but not birth control pills, which also contain estrogen), because they can still become pregnant.

Fertility

Many women are still in their childbearing years when they develop breast cancer. Of young women under thirty-five who receive chemotherapy, about half are able to get pregnant afterward.

Pregnancy following breast cancer is safe for both the mother and the baby. The hormone rush of pregnancy does not stimulate new cancer growth, and the risk of cancer recurrence is no greater in the following years in these women.

Work Issues

The return to work is an important milestone for those who have taken a partial or complete leave from their jobs during treatments. Working can give a renewed sense of self-worth and independence, as well as income and benefits. The presence of other working people itself helps restore self-esteem and self-confidence. Although feelings of self-consciousness may be present initially, these soon fade.

At work, some women are fortunate to have highly supportive employers who help ease the transition back into the job, although many don't need such assistance. Sometimes, however, wrong ideas and false fears about cancer create job-related problems that must be overcome. Frank discussions with your coworkers, as well as your employer, can often dispel such misunderstandings.

For example, it is important that everyone understands that a past episode of breast cancer, once treated, does not make a person less productive or more likely to take sick time than other workers. Studies have proven this. Likewise, it should not interfere with promotions or raises you have earned.

Some women use breast cancer as the impetus to finding a new job. However, on a job interview, you do not have to volunteer information on your health, and the employer should not ask these questions.

Uncle Sam Cares II
The federal Family and Medical Leave Act of 1993 ensures time off for workers with a major illness, providing up to twelve weeks per year of unpaid leave. An employer also cannot fire or lay off workers because of cancer or deny them health insurance or any other benefits it provides to other workers.

Life-style Changes, for the Better

During your treatments, you made some healthy changes in your daily activities, like eating a balanced diet and exercising. These changes helped you beat the cancer and to recover faster.

Now that treatments are finished, it is important to continue these healthy habits. They will help you live longer and feel better—maybe even improve your dancing or tennis game.

Diet

If you acquired a sweet—or fat—tooth while eating the high-calorie foods and snacks recommended for chemotherapy, it is time to reacquire the veggie tooth. You should eat a well-balanced, low-fat, high-fiber diet. Excess pounds only invite a whole new set of health problems.

Exercise

Many women find that, despite the nausea and loss of appetite during treatments, they actually *gained* weight. This is the revenge of all the high-cal snacks, plus side effects from some of the drugs. Some hormonal drugs, for example, do not cause nausea but can cause an increase in appetite. All of these makes the second life-style change more important.

You should continue to exercise at least as much as, if not more than, you have during treatment. This can include aerobic classes at the health club or seniors center or simple brisk walking for half an hour or more every day. Dancing, biking, tennis, swimming, running, and many other activities are beneficial as well. Breast cancer survivors have even returned to compete at the Olympics!

Regular exercise has many positive effects. The most immediate benefit is los-

> **Preventing Osteoporosis**
>
> Though estrogen-replacement therapy cannot be used for breast cancer survivors, two new drugs were recently approved that can be taken to help prevent the bone loss (osteoporosis) common to postmenopausal women. Calcitonin, in a nasal spray, and bisphosphonate, in pill form, can be prescribed by your doctor.

ing some of the weight gained during treatment, but it will also make you feel stronger and lift your spirits. Exercise also lowers your estrogen, so in theory it might reduce the chances that breast cancer could recur.

Finally, because of the breast cancer, you cannot receive the estrogen-replacement therapy that is given to many women after they reach menopause. In its place, exercise can achieve some of the same important benefits: It helps prevents bone loss (osteoporosis) and helps keep your heart healthy.

The Future

Within a few months after all treatments have ended, most women have returned to their regular routines. However, lingering feelings and anxieties are to be expected. Cancer is not something that is forgotten, but it will eventually become an experience of the past.

For some women, the recovery from breast cancer is a turning point toward a better life than before. Their priorities become clearer, their energy is redirected, and distractions are easier to ignore. Others may seize the moment to refocus and dedicate themselves to helping others—for example, volunteering to counsel other women who develop breast cancer or joining an advocacy group for women's health.

But the most important objective should be to dedicate oneself to a healthier life, enjoying friends and family a bit more, and being more accepting of life's ups and downs.

People have recovered from every type of cancer, no matter how gloomy the first reports. Yes, we're all going to die someday of something. But I plan to push that day back as far as I can, and to go out fighting whenever the time comes.

—Betty R.

It's Your Turn

1. Which doctor will you be seeing for checkups after treatments have ended?
- ❑ Surgeon
- ❑ Medical oncologist
- ❑ Your primary care physician
- ❑ Other: _____

2. Have you noticed any lingering symptoms or problems that don't seem to go away?
- ❑ Breast lump (in the same or the opposite breast?)
- ❑ Skin rash on breast
- ❑ Cough or shortness of breath
- ❑ Persistent abdominal discomfort or pain
- ❑ Dull pain in the bones
- ❑ How long have these been present?*: _____

*If any symptoms persist over several weeks, or if for any reason you are concerned, you should see your doctor.

3. If you are taking tamoxifen, have you had any unusual vaginal bleeding, spotting, or discharge or any pelvic pain or pressure?
- ❑ Yes*
- ❑ No

*This should be checked promptly by your doctor.

4. What sorts of foods do you eat in the average day?
- ❑ Basically the same as during chemotherapy
- ❑ My husband's favorite foods (he has three: pepperoni pizza, sausage pizza, and hamburger pizza)
- ❑ Balanced, low-fat, high-fiber foods*

*You should aim to eat properly, as excess weight brings other health problems.

5. How do you feel emotionally—your moods?
   - ❏ Back in the swing, making plans for the future
   - ❏ At times depressed or anxious, but it passes*
   - ❏ Still feeling tense or overwhelmed*

*Talking openly with family or other loved ones may help ease these feelings, or support groups for cancer survivors may be found at many hospitals or through the American Cancer Society. Short-term therapy with a counselor or social worker also may be an option.

6. What sort of exercise are you doing?
   - ❏ Exercise classes for breast cancer survivors (ENCORE-PLUS at the YWCA, at the hospital, others)
   - ❏ Aerobics at a health club or seniors center
   - ❏ Dance classes
   - ❏ Tennis, swimming, or running
   - ❏ Other: _____
   - ❏ None*

*Bad; start one of the above ASAP!

10

Myths and Realities: Commonly Asked Questions

 1. How can I tell if I should be concerned about a lump in my breast?

All lumps should be checked by a doctor. Most are not serious, but only the doctor can tell you this. *Sometimes a biopsy is needed to be certain.*

 2. Will I lose my breast?

Since 1990, the National Cancer Institute (NCI) has recommended that women with early-stage breast cancer be treated with breast-conserving treatment instead of mastectomy (surgery to remove the breast). Breast-conserving treatment is defined as lumpectomy (removal of the breast lump) or partial mastectomy followed by radiation therapy. Lumpectomy removes only the small piece of breast that contains the cancer, leaving a small scar and most of the breast intact.

3. Can breast cancer be cured?

Ninety-five percent of women diagnosed with early-stage breast cancer are alive at five years, the usual milestone doctors use to tell if a treatment has worked. For women with advanced-stage cancer, a cure is possible in a significant number, and the cancer can be controlled in most cases.

However, there is always the possibility of recurrence, even twenty years later. For this reason, all survivors should see their doctors for regular checkups and mammograms.

4. Is the incidence of breast cancer increasing?

From 1982 to 1987, the incidence rates for breast cancer rose by about 4 percent per year, but they have leveled off since. Most of the earlier increase is believed to be due to the wider use of screening mammography, which allows cancer to be detected in earlier stages.

5. What causes breast cancer?

No one knows for sure. And there probably isn't just one single cause. *Changes in breast cancer genes may be the most important.* The hormone estrogen, which is produced normally by women's ovaries, is thought to play a large role by making the breast cancer grow faster.

6. Can breast cancer be prevented?

There is no known way to prevent breast cancer, and 70 percent of women who get the disease have no known "risk factors." Early detection and prompt treatment are the best way to treat breast cancer successfully.

7. What about the breast cancer gene?

A test for the gene *BRCA1* is available commercially for women at high-risk and is offered to women through their doctors. *But its significance is controversial.* The gene is thought to play a role in breast cancer primarily in women under age 35, about 5 percent of the total with cancer, who are affected by hereditary or familial breast cancers.

8. Is a family history of breast cancer important?

Yes. A woman whose mother, sister, daughter, or grandmother had breast cancer has an increased risk of developing the disease. These women should be screened earlier and possibly more often. But most women with breast cancer have no family history of the disease.

9. *Does breast-feeding protect against breast cancer?*

Some studies have suggested that breast-feeding may reduce a woman's chances of developing the disease. But experts are not sure if there is any effect. A woman who breast-feeds her children can still get breast cancer.

10. How often should I have a mammogram?

The American Cancer Society recommends that after age fifty, all women get a mammogram and a clinical breast exam done by a doctor *yearly.* For women aged forty to forty-nine, a mammogram and clinical breast exam should be done at least once every year or two. Women under age 50 should talk with their doctor about how often a mammogram should be performed.

11. Can the radiation from mammograms cause breast cancer?

No. The dose of radiation to which a woman is exposed during mammography and other X ray procedures is very small and safe.

12. Does prophylactic mastectomy prevent cancer?

In a prophylactic mastectomy, the surgeon removes the breasts with no cancer, but some of the breast tissue may remain. Breast tissue extends up to the collarbone, from the chest bone around to the underarms, and down to the bottom of the ribs. A chance of developing breast cancer remains as long as there is breast tissue left in the body.

13. Can a doctor tell if a breast lump is cancerous without doing a biopsy?

Not with certainty. However, experienced doctors can tell from feeling it if a lump seems suspicious.

14. Is a mastectomy a safer option than lumpectomy and radiation?

No. The National Cancer Institute in 1990 concluded that lumpectomy followed by radiation therapy offers equally effective results as mastectomy. More recently, their conclusion was confirmed by results of the National Surgical Adjuvant Breast and Bowel Project (NSABP) protocol B-06. If cancer recurs in the breast after a lumpectomy plus radiation, mastectomy can still be done *and remains just as effective.*

15. How will I know if I need radiation treatment or chemotherapy?

Radiation therapy is always used following breast-conserving surgery. Adjuvant treatment with hormonal therapy or chemotherapy is indicated depending on the size of the tumor, lymph node status, estrogen-receptor status, and other prognostic factors, and both forms of treatment may be indicated. *However,* radiation to the chest after mastectomy is generally not indicated.

16. Will tamoxifen cause uterine cancer?

Studies have shown that in a very few cases, it can. But this usually occurs after long-term use of tamoxifen for more than five years. Therefore, most experts today recommend using tamoxifen for only two to five years. Also, uterine cancer is much more curable than breast cancer. So tamoxifen's benefits against breast cancer more than offset its small risk of causing uterine cancer.

17. Will I be able to have children after receiving chemotherapy?

About half of young women under age thirty-five who are treated with chemotherapy retain their fertility after treatment ends, and they can have safe and successful pregnancies. Women over age thirty-five to forty are less likely to remain fertile after chemotherapy.

18. My doctor asked me about joining a clinical trial. Does this mean I might get an experimental drug that might not work?

Clinical trials compare a standard treatment to a newer treatment. Before any new treatment is offered to patients, it is carefully studied in the laboratory, and it will be explained to you in detail in a process called "informed consent." Being enrolled in a clinical trial ensures that you are getting state-of-the-art care and that you will be monitored very closely.

19. How will breast cancer affect my intimate relationships?

Sexuality is an important part of everyday life. A mastectomy or lumpectomy does not interfere with your ability to experience or give pleasure. Open communication with your partner about your concern can help allay fears. A woman should not hesitate to discuss the topic of sexuality with her doctor or other members of the health care team.

20. Does it matter when during the ovulation cycle surgery is done?

Research has given conflicting results. At this time experts consider it premature to schedule surgery according to a woman's menstrual cycle.

21. Will a blood transfusion be needed during breast surgery?

Generally not for the less extensive surgeries used today to treat breast cancer. However, in breast reconstruction, the "flap" reconstruction techniques are complex and could require the use of a blood transfusion during surgery, so women might plan to donate blood beforehand for this purpose.

Appendix I
Further Information
and Support

Cancer Information Service   **800-4-CANCER** (800-422-6237)
National Cancer Institute   TTY: 800-332-8615
Bethesda, MD 20892   http://www.nci.nih.gov

A hot line staffed by information specialists trained to answer
questions about breast cancer and to help women find treatment
facilities. Free informational booklets. An excellent place to start as
well as to get information on current treatment options. In English
and Spanish.

American Cancer Society   **800-ACS-2345** (800-227-2345)
1599 Clifton Road, NE
Atlanta, GA 30329

Provides information and educational materials on breast cancer for
patients and their families. Many free publications available. It also
sponsors several programs for women with breast cancer, such as
Reach to Recovery, I Can Cope, Look Good . . . Feel Better. Call your
local ACS chapter for information.

National Alliance of Breast
Cancer Organizations (NABCO)   **800-719-9154**
9 East 37th Street, 10th floor   http://www.nabco.org
New York, NY 10016

A nonprofit network of breast cancer organizations provides advocacy as well as information, assistance, and referral to anyone with
questions about breast cancer. Publishes a comprehensive "Resource
List" ($3.00) that describes virtually all informational materials
available anywhere—very useful. Fact sheets and a newsletter
describing new developments also available.

1-800-IM-AWARE   **800-IM-AWARE** (800-462-9273)
Susan G. Komen Foundation
Occidental Tower
5005 L.B.J. Freeway, Suite 370 LB74
Dallas, TX 75244

Help line staffed by volunteers who are breast cancer survivors.
Provides support as well as information on screening, breast self-
examination, and treatment.

**Y-ME Breast Cancer
Support Program**   **800-221-2141** (English)
212 W. Van Buren Street   800-986-9595 (Spanish)
Chicago, IL 60607

Hot line staffed by volunteers who are breast cancer survivors and
who provide information and support as well as referrals to cancer
centers. Literature available. A hot line for partners is also available.

Cancer Care, Inc.   **800-813-HOPE** (800-813-4673)
1180 Avenue of the Americas   212-302-2400 (in NYC)
New York, NY 10036   http://www.cancercareinc.org

Provides support services, information, education, and referrals, as
well as professional counseling via a telephone Counseling Line and
via the Internet. Publishes the "Helping Hand" directory ($3.00) to
services and resources nationwide.

**AMC Cancer Research Center
Cancer Information Line**   **800-525-3777**
Denver, CO

Professional cancer counselors provide information and answer
questions about cancer. Free publications available.

The BMT Newsletter   **847-831-1913**
1985 Spruce Avenue   Fax: 847-831-1943
Highland Park, IL 60035

A quarterly newsletter and information for patients who are consid-
ering or have undergone bone marrow transplantation.

The Chemotherapy Foundation   **212-213-9292**
183 Madison Avenue, Suite 403
New York, NY 10016

Free booklet on chemotherapy and breast cancer available.

ENCORE-PLUS   **800-95E-PLUS** (800-953-7587)
YWCA of the United States of America
National Board
726 Broadway
New York, NY 10003

Exercise and peer-support program for women with breast cancer.
Call your local YWCA branch for information.

I Can Cope   **800-ACS-2345** (800-227-2345)
American Cancer Society

A series of eight educational classes for people with cancer and their
families, taught by local health professions and held regularly at
area hospitals. Covers diagnosis and treatment as well as day-to-day
issues of living and coping with cancer. Call your local ACS branch
for information.

Look Good . . . Feel Better   **800-395-LOOK** (800-395-5665)

A program developed by the Cosmetic, Toiletry, and Fragrance
Association Foundation in cooperation with the American Cancer
Society. Workshops to help women receiving cancer treatment learn
about skin and nail care and using makeups, cosmetics, hairstyles,
and other beauty techniques during treatment. Brochure available.
Call your local ACS chapter for information.

National Coalition for
Cancer Survivorship   **301-650-8868**
1010 Wayne Avenue, Suite 505
Silver Spring, MD 20910

A clearinghouse for information on overcoming cancer and on survivorship. Provides referrals to support services and information
sources.

National Lymphedema Network   **800-541-3259**
2211 Post Street, Suite 404   http://www.hooked.net\~lymphnet
San Francisco, CA 94115

Provides referrals, support, and information about prevention and
treatment of lymphedema.

Zeneca Breast Cancer
Patient Education Service   **800-34-LIFE4** (800-345-4334)

The manufacturer of Nolvadex (tamoxifen) will send a complimentary educational video and information on breast cancer and its treatment as well as material on tamoxifen.

Reach to Recovery   **800-ACS-2345** (800-227-2345)

Volunteers who themselves have had breast cancer visit newly diagnosed patients in the hospital and at home to provide information and support. Contact you local ACS chapter for information.

National Breast Cancer Coalition   **202-296-7477**

1707 L Street, NW, Suite 1060   http://www.natlbcc.org
Washington, DC 20036

An advocacy group.

Appendix II
Selected Readings

Breast Cancer: The Complete Guide, by Yashar Hirshaut, M.D., and Peter I. Pressman, M.D. New York: Bantam Books, 1992. 322 pages. Two breast specialists give an easy-to-follow description of diagnosis, treatment, and followup.

Breast Cancer: What Every Woman Should Know, by Rita Baron-Faust, with the physicians of the New York University Medical Center. New York: Hearst Books, 1995. 288 pages. A clear, intelligent explanation of cancer diagnosis and treatment.

The Cancer Dictionary, by Roberta Altman and Michael Sarg, M.D. New York: Facts on File, 1992. 352 pages. Helpful explanations of the many unfamiliar medical terms.

The Race Is Run One Step at a Time: My Personal Struggle and Every-woman's Guide to Taking Charge of Breast Cancer, by Nancy Brinker with Catherine McEvily Harris. Dallas, Texas: Summit Publishing Group, 1995. 270 pages. (Order from the Komen Foundation, 800-IM-AWARE.) The author's account of her sister's fight with cancer and then her own.

Dr. Susan Love's Breast Book, 2nd edition, by Susan M. Love, M.D., with Karen Lindsey. Reading, MA: Addison Wesley Publishing Co., 1995. 657 pages. An encyclopedia on the breast, how it works, and what can go wrong.

What to Do If You Get Breast Cancer, by Lydia Komarnicky, M.D., and Anne Rosenberg, M.D., with Mirian Betancourt. Boston: Little, Brown and Co., 1995. 226 pages. A practical guide to diagnosis and treatment, written by two breast specialists.

What You Need to Know About Breast Cancer, Bethesda, MD: National Cancer Institute, 1995. 44 pages. A helpful, brief outline of screening, diagnosis, and treatment.

Index

Italic page numbers refer to sidebar information and illustrations